The Exocrine Pancreas

Integrated Systems Physiology: from Molecule to Function to Disease

Editors

D. Neil Granger, *Louisiana State University Health Sciences Center-Shreveport*

Joey P. Granger, *University of Mississippi Medical Center*

Physiology is a scientific discipline devoted to understanding the functions of the body. It addresses function at multiple levels, including molecular, cellular, organ, and system. An appreciation of the processes that occur at each level is necessary to understand function in health and the dysfunction associated with disease. Homeostasis and integration are fundamental principles of physiology that account for the relative constancy of organ processes and bodily function even in the face of substantial environmental changes. This constancy results from integrative, cooperative interactions of chemical and electrical signaling processes within and between cells, organs, and systems. This eBook series on the broad field of physiology covers the major organ systems from an integrative perspective that addresses the molecular and cellular processes that contribute to homeostasis. Material on pathophysiology is also included throughout the eBooks. The state-of the-art treatises were produced by leading experts in the field of physiology. Each eBook includes stand-alone information and is intended to be of value to students, scientists, and clinicians in the biomedical sciences. Since physiological concepts are an ever-changing work-in-progress, each contributor will have the opportunity to make periodic updates of the covered material.

Published titles

(for future titles please see the Web site, www.morganclaypool.com/page/lifesci)

The Exocrine Pancreas
Stephen J. Pandol
www.morganclaypool.com

ISBN: 9781615041381   paperback

ISBN: 9781615041398   ebook

DOI: 10.4199/C00026ED1V01Y201102ISP014

A Publication in the Morgan & Claypool Publishers Life Sciences series

INTEGRATED SYSTEMS PHYSIOLOGY: FROM MOLECULE TO FUNCTION TO DISEASE #13

Book #14

Series Editors: D. Neil Granger, LSU Health Sciences Center, and Joey P. Granger, University of Mississippi Medical Center

Series ISSN

ISSN 2154-560X   print

ISSN 2154-5626   electronic

The Exocrine Pancreas

Stephen J. Pandol
University of California
Department of Veterans Affairs

INTEGRATED SYSTEMS PHYSIOLOGY:
FROM MOLECULE TO FUNCTION TO DISEASE #13

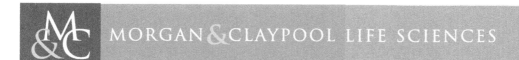

MORGAN & CLAYPOOL LIFE SCIENCES

ABSTRACT

The secretions of the exocrine pancreas provide for digestion of a meal into components that are then available for processing and absorption by the intestinal epithelium. Without the exocrine pancreas, malabsorption and malnutrition result. This chapter describes the cellular participants responsible for the secretion of digestive enzymes and fluid that in combination provide a pancreatic secretion that accomplishes the digestive functions of the gland. Key cellular participants, the acinar cell and the duct cell, are responsible for digestive enzyme and fluid secretion, respectively, of the exocrine pancreas. This chapter describes the neurohumoral pathways that mediate the pancreatic response to a meal as well as details of the cellular mechanisms that are necessary for the organ responses, including protein synthesis and transport and ion transports, and the regulation of these responses by intracellular signaling systems. Examples of pancreatic diseases resulting from dysfunction in cellular mechanisms provide emphasis of the importance of the normal physiologic mechanisms.

KEYWORDS

pancreas, secretion, digestive enzymes, acinar cell, duct cell, digestion, centroacinar cell, cholecystokinin, secretin, endoplasmic reticulum, zymogens, zymogen granule, condensing vacuole, lysosome, unfolded protein response, cystic fibrosis, trypsinogen, lipase, amylase

Contents

Introduction

The pancreas is both an exocrine organ and an endocrine organ. This chapter is devoted to the exocrine pancreas. The exocrine pancreas is responsible for secretion of digestive enzymes, ions and water into the duodenum of the gastrointestinal tract. The digestive enzymes are essential for processing foodstuffs in meals to molecular constituents that can be absorbed across the gastrointestinal surface epithelium. Although enzymes from salivary glands, the stomach and the surface epithelium of the gastrointestinal tract also participate in the digestion of a meal, the exocrine pancreas plays a central and essential role in the digestive process. With loss of exocrine pancreatic function, absorption of nutrients in markedly compromised and malnutrition ensues.

The secretion of ions and water by the exocrine pancreas is also an essential function for the exocrine pancreas. The flow of ions and water is necessary to transport the digestive enzymes from their origin in the pancreatic acinar cells to the intestine. In addition, the pH of the pancreatic secretions is alkaline due to a very high concentration of $NaHCO_3$ (up to 140 mM). At least one major function of the $NaHCO_3$ is to neutralize the acidic pH of the gastric chyme delivered to the intestine from the stomach. A neutral pH in the intestinal lumen is necessary for optimal function of digestive enzymes as well as gastrointestinal surface epithelial function.

The exocrine pancreas has been of considerable interest to physiologists and other scientists for quite some time. In fact, the first demonstration of a hormone action was in the pancreas around the turn of the 20th century [1]. The pancreas has been the major organ used to demonstrate the mechanisms of synthesis and transport for exportable proteins [2] as well as the signaling pathways involved in regulated protein secretion [3]. Also, the mechanisms that underlie the ability of the exocrine pancreas to secrete very high concentrations of $NaHCO_3$ have been of great interest to physiologists and are still debated [4–6]. This chapter presents a concise description of the current understanding of exocrine pancreatic anatomy and function with consideration of how these are affected in disease states.

Anatomy

GROSS ANATOMIC CONSIDERATIONS

In adult humans, the pancreas weighs about 80 g. The illustration in Figure 1 demonstrates the anatomical relationships between the pancreas and organs surrounding it in the abdomen. The pancreas is a retroperitoneal organ and does not have a capsule. The second and third portions of the duodenum curve around the head of the pancreas. The spleen is adjacent to the pancreatic tail. The regions of the pancreas are the head, body, tail and uncinate process (Figure 2). The distal end of the common bile duct passes through the head of the pancreas and joins the pancreatic duct entering the duodenum (Figure 1). For this reason, pathologic processes of the pancreas, such as a cancer at the head of the pancreas or swelling and/or scarring of the head of the pancreas due to pancreatitis, can lead to biliary system obstruction and injury. Because of its posterior position, the pancreas is usually protected from trauma. However, it is just anterior to the vertebral column, and severe blunt trauma to the upper abdomen as might occur from a steering wheel in an auto accident can "crush" the pancreas against the vertebral column and cause severe injury.

The arterial blood supply to the pancreas is from two major arteries supplying the abdominal organs, the celiac and superior mesenteric arteries. Because of the dual blood supply, ischemia to the pancreas from vascular obstruction is uncommon. Venous drainage of the pancreas is via the splenic vein and the superior mesenteric vein draining into the portal vein. The splenic vein runs along the body of the pancreas. Diseases, such as pancreatitis and pancreatic cancer, can involve the splenic vein leading to its thrombosis and vascular engorgement of the spleen due to the obstruction of venous blood flow.

The pancreas is innervated by both the parasympathetic and sympathetic nervous systems. The efferent parasympathetic system is contained within the branches of the vagus nerve that originates in the dorsal vagal complex (tenth cranial nerve nucleus) of the brain. The terminal branches of the vagus synapse with intrapancreatic ganglia. The postganglionic fibers innervate both exocrine and endocrine structures that are described in the next section. The sympathetic innervation originates in the lateral grey matter of the thoracic and lumbar spinal cord. The bodies of the postganglionic sympathetic neurons are located in the hepatic and celiac plexuses. The postganglionic fibers innervate blood vessels of the pancreas.

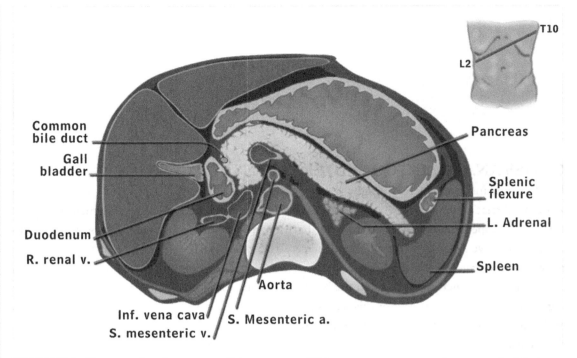

FIGURE 1: Cross-sectional anatomy of the pancreas. This cartoon represents the anatomical features of a "slice" of the abdomen at the level depicted in the upper right hand corner of the figure. Anterior to the pancreas are the stomach, colon, omentum and loops of small intestine. Posterior to the pancreas are the portal vein, inferior vena cava, aorta, superior mesenteric artery and vein, kidneys and vertebrae. The distal common bile duct passes through the head of the pancreas. Adapted from Gorelick F, Pandol, SJ, Topazian M. *Pancreatic physiology, pathophysiology, acute and chronic pancreatitis.* Gastrointestinal Teaching Project, American Gastroenterologic Association. 2003.

FUNCTIONAL ANATOMIC CONSIDERATIONS

Although this chapter is devoted to the exocrine pancreas, it is important to point out that there are important interrelationships between the endocrine (islets of Langerhans) and exocrine pancreas. The illustration in Figure 3 points out this relationship. Anatomic studies demonstrate that the blood flow from the endocrine pancreas enters the capillaries of the exocrine tissue surrounding each of the islets before entering the general circulation [7]. This "portal" system provides for the delivery of very high concentrations of hormones from the islets of Langerhans to the exocrine tissue surrounding the Islets. The hormones from the islets of Langerhans include insulin, amylin, glucagon, somatostatin and pancreatic polypeptide. Although the full significance of the effects of these hor-

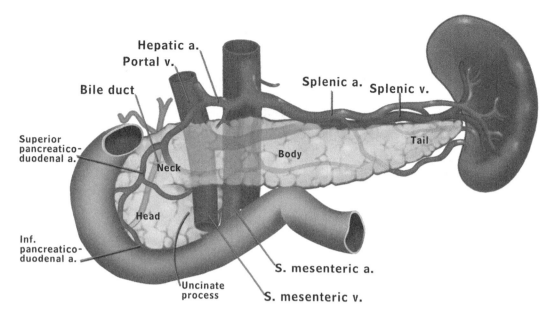

FIGURE 2: Pancreatic vascular system. The arterial blood supply to the pancreas is from two major arteries supplying the abdominal organs, the celiac and superior mesenteric arteries. The celiac artery branch supplying the pancreas is the superior pancreaticoduodenal artery. The superior mesenteric artery branch supplying the pancreas is the inferior pancreaticoduodenal artery. Venous drainage of the pancreas is via the splenic vein and the superior mesenteric vein emptying into the portal vein. Of note, the splenic vein runs along the body of the pancreas. Adapted from Gorelick F, Pandol, SJ, Topazian M. *Pancreatic physiology, pathophysiology, acute and chronic pancreatitis.* Gastrointestinal Teaching Project, American Gastroenterologic Association. 2003.

mones on the exocrine pancreas is not known, the acinar cells of the pancreas have insulin receptors that are involved in regulation of digestive enzyme synthesis of the exocrine pancreas [8–10].

The functional unit of the exocrine pancreas is composed of an acinus and its draining ductule (Figure 3). The ductal system extends from the lumen of the acinus to the duodenum. A ductule from the acinus drains into interlobular (intercalated) ducts, which in turn drain into the main pancreatic ductal system.

The acinus (from the Latin term meaning "berry in a cluster") can be spherical or tubular (Figure 3) or can have some other irregular form. The acinar cells of the acinus are specialized to synthesize, store, and secrete digestive enzymes. On the basolateral membrane are receptors for hormones and neurotransmitters that stimulate secretion of the enzymes [3]. The basal aspect of the cell

Exocrine
Acinar and duct tissue

Endocrine
Islets of Langerhans

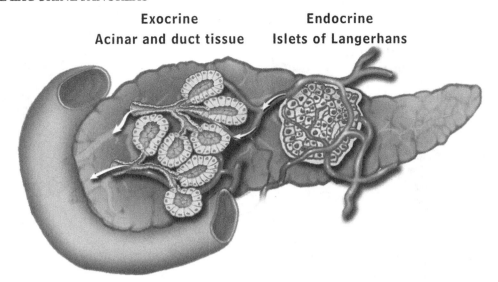

FIGURE 3: The exocrine and endocrine pancreas. The pancreas is divided into an exocrine portion (acinar and duct tissue) and an endocrine portion (islets of Langerhans). The exocrine portion, comprising 85% of the mass of the pancreas, secretes digestive enzymes, water and $NaHCO_3$ into the duodenum. The endocrine portion secretes its hormones into the blood stream. The blood flow from the endocrine pancreas passes to the exocrine pancreas before entering the general circulation. Adapted from Gorelick F, Pandol, SJ, Topazian M. *Pancreatic physiology, pathophysiology, acute and chronic pancreatitis.* Gastrointestinal Teaching Project, American Gastroenterologic Association. 2003.

contains the nucleus as well as abundant rough endoplasmic reticulum for protein synthesis (Figure 4). The apical region of the cell contains zymogen granules and store digestive enzymes. The apical surface of the acinar cell also possesses microvilli. Within the microvilli and in the cytoplasm underlying the apical plasma membrane is a filamentous actin meshwork that is involved in exocytosis of the contents of the zymogen granules [11, 12]. Secretion is into the lumen of the acinus, which is connected to the ductal system. Tight junctions between acinar cells form a band around the apical aspects of the cells and act as a barrier to prevent passage of large molecules, such as the digestive enzymes [13]. The junctional complexes also provide for the paracellular passage of water and ions.

Another intercellular connection between acinar cells is the gap junction. This specialized area of the plasma membrane between adjacent cells acts as a pore to allow small molecules (molecular weight 500 to 1000 Da) to pass between cells. The gap junction allows chemical and electrical communication between cells [3]. For example, calcium signaling is coordinated between the cells

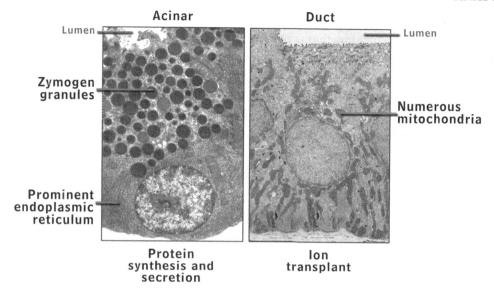

Acinar

Lumen

Zymogen
granules

Prominent
endoplasmic
reticulum

**Protein
synthesis and
secretion**

Duct

Lumen

Numerous
mitochondria

**Ion
transplant**

FIGURE 4: Ultrastructure of acinar and duct cells of the exocrine pancreas. The pancreatic acinar cell has prominent basally located rough endoplasmic reticulum for synthesis of digestive enzymes (and other proteins) and apically located zymogen granules for storage and secretion of digestive enzymes. The zymogen granules undergo exocytosis with stimulation of secretion. The secretion is into the lumen of the acinar formed by the apical surfaces of the acinar cells with their projecting microvilli. Not visualized because of the relatively low magnification are the subapical actin network, the tight junctions and the gap junctions. Pancreatic duct cells contain abundant mitochondria for energy generation needed for its ion transport functions. The ductal cells also project microvilli into the luminal space. Adapted from Gorelick F, Pandol, SJ, Topazian M. *Pancreatic physiology, pathophysiology, acute and chronic pancreatitis.* Gastrointestinal Teaching Project, American Gastroenterologic Association. 2003.

of an acinus [14, 15]. As will be discussed later in the chapter, calcium signaling represents the key pathway for digestive enzyme secretion from the acinar cell.

The duct cell epithelium consists of cells that are cuboidal to pyramidal and contain the abundant mitochondria necessary for energy products needed for ion transport (see Figure 4). Another cell that is situated at the junction of the acinus and ductule is the centroacinar cell. This cell has ductal cell characteristics but is also likely a progenitor for different cell types for the pancreas. The duct cells as well as the centroacinar cells contain carbonic anhydrase, which is important for their ability to secrete bicarbonate [5].

Another cell that is becoming important because of its role in pathologic states is the pancreatic stellate cell (PaSC) [16–21]. This is a very slender star-shaped (hence the name stellate) cell that drapes itself around the acinar and ductular structures as well as the islets of Langerhans. The role of PaSCs in normal function is probably to lay down the basement membrane to direct proper formation of the epithelial structures. Their role in pathologic states, such as chronic pancreatitis and pancreatic cancer, has been of considerable interest. In these diseases, the PaSC is transformed into a proliferating myofibroblastic cell type that synthesizes and secretes extracellular matrix proteins, proinflammatory cytokines and growth factors. These actions of the transformed PaSCs are central to the inflammatory and fibrosing pathologic processes of chronic pancreatitis and are procarcinogenic for pancreatic cancer. In fact, the myofibroblastic transformed state of the PaSC is emerging as a key participant in both the rate of growth of the cancer and the development of resistance to chemotherapy.

·   ·   ·   ·

Pancreatic Embryology and Development

The pancreas first appears at approximately 5 weeks of gestation as two outpouchings of the endodermal lining of the duodenum just distal to the forming stomach (Figure 5). The outpouchings are the ventral and dorsal pancreas. The dorsal pancreas grows more rapidly than the ventral pancreas. In addition, the ventral pancreas rotates toward the dorsal pancreas as it is "carried" by the common bile duct. Finally, the ventral and dorsal pancreas join and the ductal systems fuse so that secretions from the ventral pancreas enter the shared ductal system of the ventral pancreas and common bile duct. In the final anatomic arrangement, the head of the pancreas originates from both the dorsal pancreas and the ventral pancreas. The ventral pancreas portion is called the uncinate process. The body and tail of the pancreas originate from the dorsal pancreas.

The signaling pathways underlying the development process include the Hedgehog system, the homeobox gene Pdx1 and Notch signaling [22, 23]. Inhibition of Hedgehog signaling leads to ectopic budding of pancreatic structures in the stomach and the duodenum [24]. Pdx1 expression in the duodenum during development marks the location of pancreatic bud development [23]. Notch signaling inhibits endocrine cell differentiation and promotes exocrine cell differentiation [25]. Inhibition of Notch signaling results in marked endocrine cell expansion with blockade of exocrine cell development.

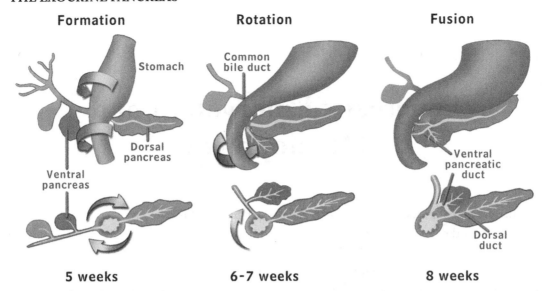

Formation   **Rotation**   **Fusion**

5 weeks   6-7 weeks   8 weeks

FIGURE 5: Pancreatic embryology. This figure demonstrates that the stomach, duodenum, biliary system, including the gallbladder, liver and pancreas are derived from closely related structures in early embryological development. The pancreas starts as two components, the ventral pancreas and the dorsal pancreas. In the process of development, the organs enlarge and the ventral pancreas together with the common bile duct rotates. Then, in most cases, the pancreatic duct from the dorsal pancreas fuses with the pancreatic duct from the ventral pancreas to form the main pancreatic duct. After fusion, the pancreatic secretions from the entire pancreas and biliary secretions gain access to the duodenum by way of the ventral pancreatic duct. Adapted from Gorelick F, Pandol, SJ, Topazian M. *Pancreatic physiology, pathophysiology, acute and chronic pancreatitis.* Gastrointestinal Teaching Project, American Gastroenterologic Association. 2003.

Digestive Enzymes

DIGESTIVE ENZYME SYNTHESIS AND TRANSPORT

The acinar cell of the exocrine pancreas has the greatest rate of protein synthesis of any mammalian organ. The acinar cell has a highly developed endoplasmic reticulum (ER) system combined with mechanisms to modify and transport newly synthesized proteins through the secretory pathway (Figure 6) [2, 26]. In addition to its functions in performing protein synthesis and processing, the ER is the major storage site for intracellular calcium, which, when released into the cytoplasm, is the mediator of regulated secretion of stored digestive enzymes into the pancreatic ductal system [27].

Each protein synthesized in the ER must undergo specific secondary modifications as well as folding in order for it to be properly transported to destination organelles, such as Golgi, zymogen granule (storage for the digestive enzymes) and lysosome or membrane sites. The zymogen granule stores digestive enzymes and are released by exocytosis with neurohumoral stimulation with a meal as described below. Also, the systems for both protein synthesis and processing must be able to adapt because of the variation in the demand for protein synthesis as a function of diet and because protein processing in the ER could be adversely affected by environmental factors, such as alcohol, smoking, altered metabolism and xenobiotics.

Synthesis of digestive enzymes takes place in the internal space of the rough endoplasmic reticulum (RER) (Figure 7). The mechanism for translation of the cell's messenger RNA (mRNA) into exportable protein is explained by the signal hypothesis [28, 29]. The main feature of the hypothesis is that ribosomal subunits attach to mRNA and initiate synthesis of a hydrophobic "signal" sequence on the NH_2-terminal of nascent proteins. This complex then attaches to the outer surface of the endoplasmic reticulum, and the signal sequence targets the protein being synthesized into the lumen of the RER.

Newly synthesized proteins can undergo modifications in the endoplasmic reticulum, including disulfide bridge formation, phosphorylation, sulfation and glycosylation. Conformational changes resulting in tertiary and quaternary structures of the protein also take place in the endoplasmic reticulum. Processed proteins from the endoplasmic reticulum are transported to the Golgi complex where further posttranslational modification (glycosylation) and concentration occur [30].

The Golgi complex also serves the important function of sorting and targeting newly synthesized proteins into various cell compartments (Figure 6). Digestive enzymes are transported to the

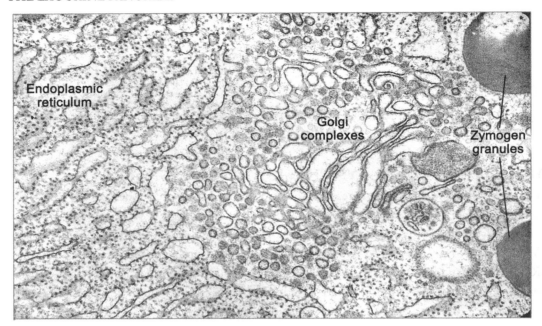

FIGURE 6: Electron micrograph of the pancreatic acinar cell. This electron micrograph shows the key cellular structures involved in synthesis, processing and storage of digestive enzymes. On the left is the rough endoplasmic reticulum; in the middle is the Golgi complex; and on the right are zymogen granules. Adapted from Gorelick F, Pandol, SJ, Topazian M. *Pancreatic physiology, pathophysiology, acute and chronic pancreatitis.* Gastrointestinal Teaching Project, American Gastroenterologic Association. 2003.

zymogen granules [30]. Lysosomal hydrolases are sorted to the lysosome [31]. For this lysosomal pathway, mannose-6-phosphate groups are added to oligosaccharide chains on the protein during its presence in the *cis*-Golgi complex. The mannose-6-phosphate groups serve as a recognition site for a specific receptor. The interaction of the lysosomal enzyme mannose-6-phosphate with its receptor leads to formation of vesicles that transport this complex to the lysosome, delivering the enzyme. In the lysosome, the enzyme dissociates from the receptor, which in turn cycles back to the Golgi complex.

Secretion of the digestive enzymes occurs by exocytosis. Exocytosis consists of movement of the secretory granule to the apical surface, the recognition of a plasma membrane site for fusion, and the fission of the granule membrane/plasma membrane site after fusion [2, 32]. Roles for actin–myosin, SNARE (soluble *N*-ethylmaleimide-sensitive factor attachment protein [SNAP] receptor) proteins and guanosine triphosphate (GTP)-binding proteins have been demonstrated to participate in the exocytosis processes [33–40]. Intracellular signals generated by agonist receptors as discussed below interact with these entities to mediate digestive enzyme secretion via exocytosis of zymogen granules.

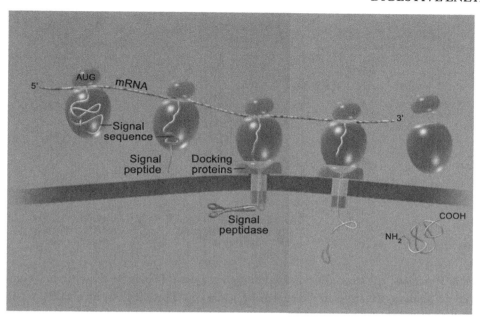

FIGURE 7: The signal hypothesis mechanism of protein synthesis. The endoplasmic reticulum is the site of new protein synthesis. The mechanism of protein synthesis is initiated with the attachment of a messenger RNA (mRNA) to ribosomal subunits. As illustrated, a single mRNA can be processed sequentially by several ribosomal units yielding several protein copies for each mRNA. The association of several ribosomal subunits to an mRNA is called a polysome. The 5′ terminal end of each mRNA is the same signal codon leading to the synthesis of a signal sequence. This signal sequence promotes attachment of the ribosomal unit to docking proteins in the ER membrane. Then protein synthesis continues with the nascent protein passing into the cisternal space of the ER. The transport of the nascent protein across the ER membrane is facilitated by the hydrophobic properties of the signal sequence. After the protein has been directed to the cisternal space of the ER, the signal is cleaved from the protein by signal peptidase. This cleavage entraps the newly synthesized protein in the ER cisternal space. Adapted from Gorelick F, Pandol, SJ, Topazian M. *Pancreatic physiology, pathophysiology, acute and chronic pancreatitis.* Gastrointestinal Teaching Project, American Gastroenterologic Association. 2003.

ENVIRONMENTAL AND GENETIC STRESSORS AND THE SECRETORY PATHWAY

As indicated above, proteins enter the ER as unfolded polypeptides that require further processing for activation and targeting to the appropriate organelle or membrane site. In this transport, the ER and other organelles along the secretory pathway are faced with several challenges in completing these functions with high fidelity. Figure 8 illustrates many of these challenges, which are often referred to as ER stress in many organs including the exocrine pancreas. At the bottom of the

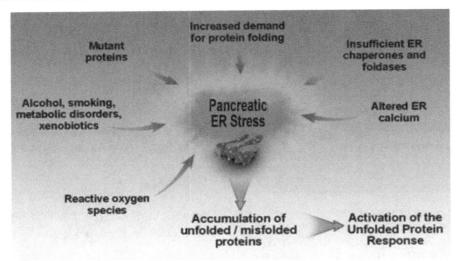

FIGURE 8: Pancreatic ER stress the unfolded protein response. The figure shows several types of factors that could promote ER stress in the pancreatic acinar cell. These include increased protein folding demand, insufficient ER chaperone and foldase function, mutant proteins, alcohol, smoking, metabolic disorders, xenobiotics, reactive oxygen species and altered ER calcium. These stresses lead to unfolded and misfolded proteins, which, in turn, activates the unfolded protein response in an attempt to adapt cellular machinery to the stress.

figure, the unfolded protein response (UPR) that results from the stressors and mediates an adaptive response so that the exocrine pancreas can adjust its machinery to the effects of the stressors and proceed with normal synthetic and transport functions is indicated. The types of both genetic and environmental insults depicted here are the ones that are known to be ER stressors in general [41]. For the exocrine pancreas, in particular, the machinery must adapt to increased protein loads requiring processing during and after a meal as the pancreas replenishes its stores of digestive enzymes. This increased load would require synthesis of chaperones and foldases, as well as upregulation of the systems involved in degradation of unfolded and misfolded proteins. The quality control system to degrade these unusable proteins called ER-associated protein degradation (ERAD) is required to rid the cell from accumulation of permanently misfolded and unfolded proteins that are toxic to the cell.

There are several genetic and environmental stressors illustrated in Figure 8 that occur in the pancreas that are likely ER stressors requiring the acinar cell to activate its adaptive UPR or face the possibility of cellular pathologies. For example, mutations in key protease digestive enzymes are known to lead to chronic forms of pancreatitis and increased rate of pancreatic cancer [42]. A recent report [43], in fact, demonstrates that a mutation in human cationic trypsinogen causes ER stress in pancreatic cells suggesting that the chronic form of pancreatitis occurring in patients with this mutation occurs because the UPR is insufficiently robust to adjust to the ER stress caused by the mutation.

Other stressors encountered by the exocrine pancreatic acinar cell UPR and shown in Figure 8 include alcohol, smoking, metabolic disorders and xenobiotics as well as reactive oxygen species (ROS). Except for information on the genetic mutation discussed above and recent work on alcohol abuse [44], there is little information on these factors affecting the pancreas and ER stress and whether pathology results from an insufficiently robust UPR. Alcohol abuse and smoking are key risk factors in the epidemiology of the major diseases of the exocrine pancreas, pancreatitis and pancreatic cancer [17, 45, 46]. Recent epidemiologic studies demonstrate that smoking accelerates the development of pancreatitis in alcoholic patients and may have an additive or multiplicative effect when combined with alcohol to cause pancreatitis [45, 47]. An important and unexplained observation is that only a small proportion of heavy drinkers/smokers develop pancreatic diseases [48]. Although the reason for lack of development of pathology in the majority of those who drink and smoke is unknown, it is likely that the exocrine pancreas adapts to the environmental stressors with a robust UPR preventing cellular pathology in most individuals. Inability to adapt completely may lead to cellular pathologies.

EXOCRINE PANCREATIC UPR ADAPTIVE RESPONSE

The adaptive UPR has three major functions [41, 49–52]. These include: 1) an upregulation of the expression and function of chaperones and foldases to augment the folding and export capacity of the ER; 2) activation of the ER-associated protein degradation (ERAD) system to rid the ER of accumulated unfolded and misfolded proteins; and 3) a global reduction in translation of mRNA to decrease the processing demand for newly synthesized proteins. Under severe and prolonged stress that exceeds to its adaptive capacity, the UPR can initiate cell death programs.

Figure 9 presents an overview of UPR, showing that there are three main sensor–transducers located in the membrane of the ER [41, 49]. They are inositol-requiring protein-1 (IRE1), activating transcription factor-6 (ATF6) and protein kinase RNA (PKR)-like ER kinase (PERK). In each case, the transmembrane sensor–transducer measures the ER luminal environment as well as the folding status of the proteins there and transmits this information across the ER membrane. In some cases, the transmembrane sensor–transducer is "silenced" by binding of an ER chaperone called immunoglobulin-binding protein (BiP) to its luminal domain. ER stress unfolded and misfolded proteins compete for binding BiP, resulting in removing its "silencing" effect and in activation of the sensor. This represents one way for activation of sensor–transducers. However, there are likely many other mechanisms that have yet to be determined.

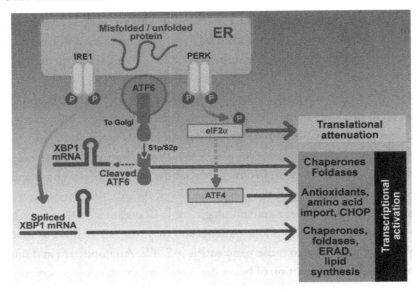

FIGURE 9: The participants of the unfolded protein response. The figure shows the three main sensor/transducers of the unfolded response, inositol-requiring protein-1 (IRE1), activating transcription factor-6 (ATF6) and protein kinase RNA (PKR)-like ER kinase (PERK). The details of the pathways and responses activated by the senor/transducers are described in detail in the accompanying text. Adapted from Rutkowski and Kaufman. Trends Biochem Sci 2007;32:469–76.

Activation of the IRE1sensor–transducer initiates a response to increase the expression of ER chaperones and foldases to assist in protein folding and transport (Figure 9). The mechanism of sensing stress involves IRE1 homodimerization and *trans*-autophosphorylation to activate a specific RNAse activity that it carries. IRE1 RNAse cleaves the mRNA for unspliced X-box binding protein1 (XBP1). Activated IRE1 removes a 26-nucleotide intron from XBP1 resulting in an mRNA that translates into a potent transcription factor called spliced XBP1 (XBP1-S) [53–55]. XBP1-S, in turn, binds to ER stress element (ERSE) and the UPR element (UPRE) DNA binding sites to upregulate many UPR target genes, such as the chaperones BiP and GRP94 and the gene encoding XBP1-U [53–56]. This ability to increase transcription of XBP1 leads to more substrates for expression of the XBP1-S transcription factor, thus, augmenting this protective response. The IRE1/XBP1 pathway also leads to increased expression of foldases, such as protein disulfide isomerase (PDI), enzymes for lipid synthesis for expanding the ER membrane and ER capacity, components of the ER-associated degradation (ERAD), all protective mechanisms to adapt the system to the stress [56].

ATF6 is another ER transmembrane protein that responds to ER stress (Figure 9). The C-terminal luminal domain is sensitive to ER stress, while the N-terminal cytoplasmic domain contains a DNA transcription-activating domain. Release of BiP binding that occurs as BiP alternatively binds to unfolded proteins during ER stress allows ATF6 transport to the Golgi compartment where it is cleaved by site-1 and site-2 proteases (sp1/sp2) to a 50–60 kDa fragment that migrates to the nucleus to activate transcription of XBP1 and other UPR target genes [57]. This shows a coordinated effort between the IRE1 and ATF6 pathways to mediate an adaptive ER protective response utilizing XBP1.

As indicated, XBP1-S is a potent transcription activator for many UPR target genes including the molecular chaperone BiP. The increased expression would allow more BiP available to inactivate the ER sensors. Thus, BiP acts as a luminal sensor of unfolded proteins as well as the regulator of mechanisms to initiate the protective UPR, including the production of sufficient BiP to attenuate an ER stress response.

PERK plays a key role in adjusting the cell to ER stress by causing a significant attenuation of general protein synthesis (Figure 9). The activation of PERK by autophosphorylation (Thr^{980}) leads to its phosphorylation of the alpha subunit of the eukaryotic translation initiation factor-2α (eIF-2α) [57, 58]. The nonphosphorylated form of eIF-2α in its GTP-bound form is essential for translation initiation because it recruits the first tRNA ($tRNA^{MET}$) to the ribosomal subunits to start translation of the attached mRNA. Phosphorylation of eIF2α at Ser51 by PERK blocks eIF2α-mediated initiation, resulting in a general inhibition of protein synthesis. Cells with genetic deletion of PERK or cells containing eIF2α with position 51 containing alanine instead of serine to prevent phosphorylation do not attenuate protein synthesis with ER stress [59, 60]. As a consequence, cells are more sensitive to ER stress. This shows that general inhibition of protein synthesis by the PERK signaling pathway is another key way where the pancreas can adapt to stress responses. Persistent phosphorylation of eIF2α leads to specific translational upregulation of activating transcription factor 4 (ATF4) that targets genes involved in antioxidant effects including synthesis of glutathione [61]. ATF4 also upregulates the expression of the transcription factor C/EBP homologous protein (CHOP) which induces apoptosis [62]. This last pathway shows how a high level of sustained ER stress can lead to pathologic consequences that results when the adaptive responses are insufficiently robust to attenuate the stress posed on the protein synthesis and transport mechanisms.

ENVIRONMENTAL STRESS AND DISEASES OF THE EXOCRINE PANCREAS

The most common diseases of the exocrine pancreas are pancreatitis and pancreatic cancer. Alcohol abuse and smoking are key risk factors in the epidemiology of both diseases [17, 45, 46]. In the case of alcohol abuse, the increased risk for pancreatic cancer occurs largely through the effect of alcohol abuse causing chronic forms of pancreatitis [63]. Smoking also contributes to the development of pancreatitis and is a major risk factor for pancreatic cancer independent of pancreatitis [17, 46, 63]. Recent epidemiologic studies demonstrate that smoking accelerates the development of pancreatitis in alcoholic patients and may have an additive or multiplicative effect when combined with alcohol to cause pancreatitis [45, 47]. The mechanisms underlying the effects of alcohol and smoking on the development of pancreatic diseases are incompletely understood. An important and unexplained observation is that only a small proportion of heavy drinkers/smokers develop pancreatic diseases [48]. Although the reason for lack of development of pathology in the majority of those who drink and smoke is unknown, we hypothesize that an adaptive UPR is sufficiently robust in most individuals to prevent pathology.

DIGESTIVE ENZYMES AND THEIR FUNCTIONS

The human pancreas has the largest capacity for protein synthesis of any organ in the human body. Much of the capacity is devoted to synthesis of the digestive enzymes that are secreted in the intestinal lumen. Table 1 lists the major proteolytic, amylolytic, lipolytic and nuclease digestive enzymes [64–66]. Some of the enzymes are present in more than one form (e.g., cationic trypsinogen, anionic trypsinogen and mesotrypsinogen). Further, they are capable of digesting the cell and causing significant damage. There are mechanisms to prevent these enzymes from potentially digesting the pancreas including storage and packing in acidic zymogen granules to inhibit activity; and synthesis and storage as inactive precursor forms. The lists in Table 1 show some of the enzymes that are stored in the pancreas before secretion as inactive proenzymes. These proenzymes are activated when they enter the duodenum. As illustrated in Figure 10, activation of these enzymes takes place in the surface of the duodenal lumen, where a brush-border glycoprotein peptidase, enteroki-

TABLE 1: Digestive proenzymes and enzymes in the pancreas. Digestive enzymes are stored in the pancreas as either inactive proenzyme forms or active enzymes.

PROENZYMES	ENZYMES
Trypsinogens (1, 2, 3)	
Chymotrypsinogen (A, B)	α-Amylase
Procarboxypeptidase A (1, 2)	Lipase
Procarboxypeptidase B (1, 2)	DNase
Prophospholipase (I, II)	RNase
Proelastase	
Mesotrypsin	

nase, activates trypsinogen by removing (by hydrolysis) an N-terminal hexapeptide fragment of the molecule (Val–Asp–Asp–Asp–Asp–Lys) [65–67]. The active form, trypsin, then catalyzes the activation of the other inactive proenzymes. Of note, many key digestive enzymes, such as α-amylase and lipase, are present in the pancreas in their active forms (Table 1). Presumably, these enzymes would not cause pancreatic cellular damage if released into the pancreatic cell/tissue because there is no starch, glycogen or triglyceride substrate for these enzymes in pancreatic tissue.

Another mechanism that the exocrine pancreas utilizes to prevent intracellular activation involves the synthesis and incorporation of a trypsin inhibitor (pancreatic secretory trypsin inhibitor [PSTI]) into the secretory pathway and zymogen granule. PSTI is a 56-amino acid peptide that inactivates trypsin by forming a relatively stable complex with the enzyme near its catalytic site [68]. The function of the inhibitor is to inactivate trypsins that are formed autocatalytically in the pancreas or pancreatic juice, thus, preventing pancreatic digestion and resulting disorders, such as pancreatitis [69, 70]. In the following paragraphs are descriptions of the functions of the major digestive enzymes.

Amylase is secreted by both the pancreas and salivary glands, differing in molecular weight, carbohydrate content and electrophoretic mobility [71]. However, they have identical enzyme

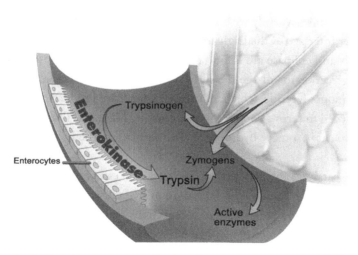

FIGURE 10: Intestinal digestive enzyme activation. Inactive proenzymes called zymogens enter the duodenum where enterokinase which is attached to the intestinal surface ally enzymatic leaves trypsinogen activating it to trypsin. Trypsin, in turn, converts zymogens including trypsinogen itself to their activated enzyme forms through enzymatic cleavage. Adapted from Gorelick F, Pandol, SJ, Topazian M. *Pancreatic physiology, pathophysiology, acute and chronic pancreatitis.* Gastrointestinal Teaching Project, American Gastroenterologic Association. 2003.

activities. Salivary amylase initiates digestion in the mouth and may account for a significant portion of starch and glycogen digestion because it is transported with the meal into the stomach and small intestine, where it continues to have activity. Optimal enzyme activity occurs at neutral pH. During a meal, gastric pH can approach neutrality despite gastric acid secretion because of the buffering from molecules in the meal as well as alkaline secretions from the salivary glands and gastric mucus. Salivary amylase can contribute up to 50% of starch and glycogen digestion while pancreatic amylase contributes the remainder. The action of both salivary and pancreatic amylase is to hydrolyze 1,4-glycoside linkages at every other junction between carbon 1 and oxygen. The products of amylase digestion are maltose and maltotriose (2- and 3-α-1,4-linked molecules, respectively) and α-dextrins containing 1,6-glycosidic linkages because 1,6-glycosidic linkages in starch cannot be hydrolyzed by amylase. The brush-border enzymes complete the hydrolysis of the products of amylase digestion to glucose. The final product, glucose, is transported across the intestinal absorptive epithelial cell by a Na^+-coupled transport [72, 73].

Lipases are secreted mainly by the pancreas in contrast to amylase where there is a significant salivary contribution. There are lingual and gastric lipases but these contribute to fat digestion in only a minor fashion. Major lipases secreted by the pancreas are lipase (or triglyceride lipase) and prophospholipases (Table 1).

Pancreatic lipase hydrolyzes a triglyceride molecule to two fatty acid molecules released from carbons 1 and 3 and a monoglyceride with a fatty acid esterified to glycerol at carbon 2 [74]. Lipase binds to the oil/water interface of the triglyceride oil droplet, where it acts to hydrolyze the triglyceride. Both bile acids and colipase are important for the full activity of lipase. Bile acids aid in the emulsification of triglyceride to enlarge the surface area for lipase to act on, and they form micelles with fatty acids and monoglyceride, which, in turn, remove these products from the oil/water interface. Colipase is believed to form a complex with lipase and bile salts. This ternary complex anchors lipase and allows it to act in a more hydrophilic environment on the hydrophobic surface of the oil droplet.

Phospholipase catalyzes the hydrolysis of the fatty acid ester linkage at carbon 2 of phosphatidylcholine [66]. This cleavage leads to the formation of free fatty acid and lysophosphatidylcholine.

Proteases secreted by the pancreas are generally divided into two groups—the endopeptidases and the exopeptidases (Figure 11). All are stored and secreted from the pancreas as inactive proforms that are activated in the duodenum by trypsin. Trypsin, chymotrypsin and elastase are endopeptidases that cleave specific peptide bonds adjacent to specific amino acids within a protein. Exopeptidases include carboxypeptidases that cleave peptide bonds at the carboxyl terminus of proteins.

Importantly, the combined actions of the pancreatic proteases and pepsin from the stomach result in the formation of oligopeptides and free amino acids. The oligopeptides are further di-

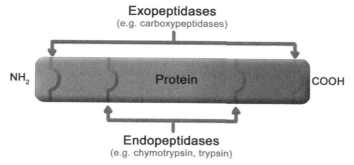

FIGURE 11: Classification of proteases. This graphic presents two major types of proteases, the exopeptidases that cleave peptide bonds releasing one amino acid at a time from the NH_2 or COOH terminal ends of a protein; and the endopeptidases that cleave peptide bonds internally in a protein at specific sites. Examples of exopeptidases are carboxypeptidases that cleave peptide bonds from COOH terminal of a protein. Examples of endopeptidases are chymotrypsin and trypsin. Trypsin cleavage is specific for the peptide bonds after arginine and lysine residues in the protein whereas chymotrypsin specifically cleaves peptide bonds after aromatic amino acids. Adapted from Gorelick F, Pandol, SJ, Topazian M. *Pancreatic physiology, pathophysiology, acute and chronic pancreatitis.* Gastrointestinal Teaching Project, American Gastroenterologic Association. 2003.

gested by brush-border enzymes on the lumenal surface of the small intestine. Both free amino acids and oligopeptides are transported across the intestinal mucosa by a group of Na^+- and H^+-coupled transporters [75]. It is interesting that only certain amino acids (mostly essential amino acids) and oligopeptides can be measured in the lumen during digestion, indicating that the combined action of the proteases is not random and that the products result from the combined specificities of the individual proteases. These amino acids have greater effects on stimulating pancreatic secretion, inhibiting gastric emptying, regulating small bowel motility and causing satiety. Thus, the specific pattern of protease actions leads to the physiologic regulation of several organs in the gastrointestinal tract.

REGULATION OF DIGESTIVE ENZYME SYNTHESIS

The mechanisms involved in regulating expression of digestive enzymes in the exocrine pancreas have been partially elucidated. The investigations have addressed the following two questions: First, what accounts for the specific expression of digestive enzymes in the pancreas? Second, how do alterations in dietary nutrients change the synthesis of specific digestive enzymes? Genes for digestive enzymes, such as amylase, chymotrypsin and elastase, contain enhancer regions in their 5′ flanking nucleotide sequences that regulate the transcription of their mRNAs, termed the pancreas consensus element (PCE) [76–78]. A transcription factor, PTF-1, is present selectively in the exocrine pancreas, binds to this region and is essential for expression of these digestive enzymes [77–82]. Thus, PTF-1 represents at least one of the differentiation-regulated factors that accounts for digestive enzyme expression in the pancreas.

Numerous studies have demonstrated that the relative synthesis rates of specific digestive enzymes change as a function of dietary intake. For example, a carbohydrate-rich diet results in an increase in synthesis of amylase and a decrease in that of chymotrypsinogen [83]; a lipid-rich diet enhances lipase expression [84]; and an alcohol-rich diet decreases amylase expression [85]. The mechanisms responsible for this adaptation are only partially understood. The regulation occurs at the level of gene transcription in many of these conditions [85]. Several studies have also demonstrated that amylase gene expression is regulated by both insulin and diet [83].

STIMULATION OF DIGESTIVE ENZYME SECRETION FROM THE ACINAR CELL

Digestive enzymes synthesized and stored in the zymogen granule are available for transport and release into the lumen of the pancreatic acinus and transport through the pancreatic ductal system into the intestine. The transport and release of zymogen granule contents occurs through exocytosis [2]. *In vitro* preparations of acinar cells from the pancreas of small animals have been used extensively to determine the mechanisms of regulation of exocytosis and digestive enzyme secretion (Figure 12). The results using animal pancreatic tissue have been confirmed in part using preparations of human pancreatic acinar cells [86].

Functional receptors that mediate digestive enzyme secretion have been identified for cholecystokinin (CCK), acetylcholine, gastrin-releasing peptide (GRP), substance P, vasoactive intestinal peptide (VIP) and secretin in preparations of pancreatic acinar cells from several species by measuring responses to ligands specific for the receptors and using radiolabelled ligand binding studies [87]. Furthermore, the molecular structure for each of these receptor types has been elucidated from cloning and sequencing [88]. Each is a G-protein-coupled receptor (GPCR) with seven hydrophobic domains believed to be membrane-spanning segments. The receptors are on the basolateral plasma membrane of the acinar cell.

The GPCRs on the acinar cells have been divided into two groups according to their mechanisms of stimulating secretion (Figure 12). In one category are GPCRs for each the neurotransmitter VIP and the hormone secretin. The interaction of each of these agonists with their specific GPCRs on acinar cells leads to activation of adenylate cyclase and a rise in cellular cAMP, which in turn activates enzyme secretion through cAMP-dependent protein kinase A [89]. In the other group are GPCRs for the neurotransmitter acetylcholine, GRP and substance P and the hormone CCK. Interaction of each agonist in this group with its specific GPCR causes secretion through the phosphoinositide-calcium signaling system [3, 27]. The agonist–receptor interaction for these re-

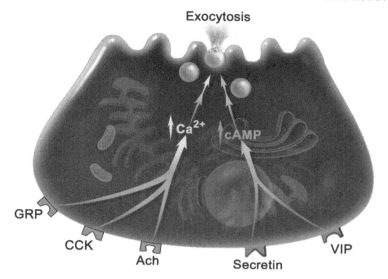

FIGURE 12: Regulation of exocytosis. Digestive enzymes are stored in zymogen granules at the apical surface of the acinar cell. Regulated secretion occurs through exocytosis stimulated by neurohumoral agents. These agents include gastrin-releasing peptide (GRP), cholecystokinin (CCK), acetylcholine (Ach), secretin and vasoactive intestinal polypeptide (VIP). Each acts to mediate secretion through interacting with its specific receptor. For example, specific interaction of CCK with its receptor (CCK1 receptor) leads to activation of intracellular signaling systems that mediate the exocytosis response. Interactions of GRP, CCK and Ach with their receptors leads to changes in intracellular which, in turn, mediates exocytosis. On the other hand, secretin and VIP increase intracellular cAMP which, in turn, mediates the exocytosis response. Of note, an increase in both calcium and cAMP simultaneously results in synergistic response. That is, the response with both is greater than the expected additive effect. Adapted from Gorelick F, Pandol, SJ, Topazian M. *Pancreatic physiology, pathophysiology, acute and chronic pancreatitis.* Gastrointestinal Teaching Project, American Gastroenterologic Association. 2003.

ceptors leads to a phospholipase C-mediated hydrolysis of phosphatidylinositol 4,5-bisphosphate to 1,2-diacylglycerol and inositol 1,4,5-triphosphate (IP_3). IP_3, in turn, releases calcium from endoplasmic reticulum stores. The calcium release into the cytosol causes a rapid rise in the concentration of free calcium ($[Ca^{+2}]_i$) that is necessary for the secretory response. With physiologic concentrations of agonists, the increase in $[Ca^{+2}]_i$ initiates in the apical area of acinar cell in the vicinity of the zymogen granules followed by a propagated "wave" toward the basolateral area of the cell [90–93]. Also, the increases in $[Ca^{+2}]_i$ are transient giving an oscillatory pattern. Each spike in $[Ca^{+2}]_i$ leads to a "burst" in zymogen granule exocytosis and secretion. Calcium release into the cytosol is also mediated by ryanodine receptors and signals interacting with the ryanodine receptor, such as calcium and fatty acid-coenzyme A esters [94]. Other intracellular signaling molecules involved in intracellular calcium release are cyclic adenosine diphosphate (ADP)-ribose and nicotinic acid adenine dinucleotide phosphate (NAADP) [27]. These messengers are involved in propagating and regulating the "waves" and "oscillations" that are essential to the physiologic calcium signaling that mediates secretion.

The mechanisms by which increases in $[Ca^{+2}]_i$ mediate secretion are not established but involve calmodulin-dependent protein kinases and actin–myosin interactions, SNARE proteins and guanosine triphosphate-binding proteins, as discussed earlier [87]. The continued stimulation of enzyme secretion by these agents also depends on the influx of extracellular calcium [95]. This influx is regulated by changes in nitric oxide and cyclic guanosine monophosphate (cGMP) [96]. The components of the plasma membrane calcium influx channel have been determined and involved [97, 98, 99].

The digestive enzyme secretory response may also be regulated by 1,2-diacylglycerol, protein kinase C and arachidonic acid [100, 101]. Specific phosphorylations and dephosphorylations of cellular proteins also occur with both cAMP agonists and calcium-phosphoinositide agonists [3]. The exact roles of these events in secretion are not established.

The enzyme secretory response of the acinar cell to a combination of an agonist that acts through cAMP and an agonist that acts through changes in calcium is greater than the sum of the individual responses. An example of such a combination would be VIP or secretin with acetylcholine. The exact mechanism of this potentiated response is not known, but it functions physiologically so that significant quantities of secretion occur with a combination of small increases in individual agonists.

Water and Ion Secretion from the Pancreatic Ductal System

FLOW AND ION CONCENTRATIONS OF PANCREATIC FLUID

Water and ions sodium, potassium, chloride and bicarbonate are the main inorganic constituents of pancreatic secretion (Figure 13). These constituents and their flow during a meal are necessary for transporting pancreatic enzymes secreted from the acinar cell to the intestinal lumen. As discussed below, disorders of water and ion secretion lead to pancreatic exocrine tissue damage and exocrine failure as occurs in cystic fibrosis. Another key function of pancreatic water and ion secretion is

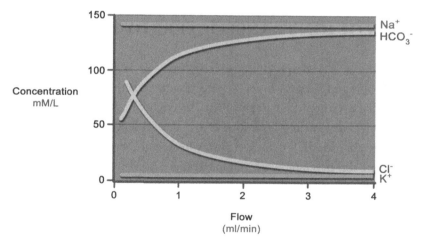

FIGURE 13: Concentrations of ions in pancreatic secretions. The graph illustrates that with increasing stimulation of pancreatic flow (as would occur during a meal with secretin stimulation) there are marked changes in the concentrations of ions in the fluid marked by a dramatic increase in HCO_3^- and a simultaneous decrease in Cl^- for HCO_3^-. There is no change in the concentration of Na^+ or K^+ or total ion concentration. Adapted from Gorelick F, Pandol, SJ, Topazian M. *Pancreatic physiology, pathophysiology, acute and chronic pancreatitis.* Gastrointestinal Teaching Project, American Gastroenterologic Association. 2003.

neutralization of gastric acid emptied into the duodenum. The neutralization of gastric acid is necessary because the pancreatic enzymes have optimal activity at neutral pH. At the acid pH of gastric secretions, pancreatic digestive enzymes are ineffective in digesting a meal.

As discussed in the Regulation of Whole-Organ Pancreatic Secretion section, the regulation of water and ion secretions is largely mediated by the hormone secretin and the neurotransmitter acetylcholine stimulation of the pancreatic ductal cell. Of note, acinar cell secretion of digestive enzymes is accompanied by a low-volume secretion isotonic with plasma with ion concentrations of sodium, potassium, chloride and bicarbonate that are similar to those in plasma. Ductal secretion during the intestinal phase of the meal is much greater in volume than acinar secretion and is clear, colorless, alkaline and isotonic with plasma. The flow rate increases from an average rate of 0.2 or 0.3 mL/min in the resting (interdigestive) state to 4.0 mL/min during stimulation of a meal. The total daily volume of secretion is about 2.5 L. The major feature of secretin- and acetylcholine-stimulated ductal secretion in addition to the increase in volume is an increase in bicarbonate concentration with a reciprocal decrease in chloride concentration (Figure 13). The exocrine pancreatic duct is unique in its ability to secrete a fluid with bicarbonate concentrations as great as 140 mM [4–6]. The ductular epithelium and the centroacinar cell are enriched in the enzyme carbonic anhydrase which facilities the formation of bicarbonate from CO_2 and H_2O [102, 103].

REGULATION OF ION TRANSPORTERS OF THE PANCREATIC DUCT CELL

Secretin stimulates ductal secretion by binding to its receptor on the ductal cell and probably the centroacinar cell. Binding of secretin to its receptor results in activating adenylate cyclase and increasing cyclic adenosine monophosphate (cAMP). Acetylcholine does so by binding to its receptor and raising intracellular calcium concentrations [4–6]. The initial events involve cAMP-dependent and Ca^{+2}-dependent chloride (Cl^-) channel activation on the luminal membrane as well as K^+ channel activation on the basolateral membrane (Figure 14) [4–6]. The cAMP-dependent Cl^- channel is the cystic fibrosis transmembrane conductance regulator (CFTR) which has been demonstrated to be located on the apical surface of ductal epithelium in human pancreas [104]. The activation of both channels by cAMP leads to Cl^- secretion into the lumen. The higher chloride concentration in the lumen is coupled to a Cl^-/HCO_3^- antiport, resulting in an exchange of Cl^- for HCO_3^- in the lumen. Newer evidence also suggests a HCO_3^- channel on the apical surface involved in HCO_3^- secretion and that this HCO_3^- conductance includes CFTR [4–6, 105]. On the basolateral surface of the duct cell are a Na^+- and H^+-antiport and a Na^+/HCO_3^- cotransport as well as ATPases (Na^+/K^+-ATPase, H^+-ATPase) and K^+ channels. In combination, these transporters facilitate HCO_3^- secretion at the apical surface as well as maintain intracellular pH [106]. For example, the K^+ channels activated by cAMP and Ca^{+2} and the Na^+/K^+-ATPase create an intracel-

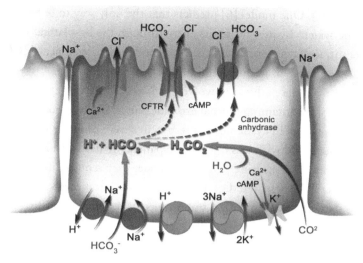

FIGURE 14: The transporters of the pancreatic duct cell. The central purpose of the pancreatic ductal system is to secrete a large volume of water with a concentration of about 140 mM $NaHCO_3$. The pancreatic duct cell is equipped with transporters and mechanisms to accomplish this task. First of all, delivery of large amounts of HCO_3^- is accomplished by two mechanisms. In one large amounts of carbonic anhydrase in ductal cells converts CO_2 rapidly to HCO_3^- and H^+. A second mechanism involves a Na^+ and HCO_3^- cotransport on the basolateral surface of the cell. The secretion is mediated by cAMP and Ca^{2+} intracellular signaling activated by secretin and acetylcholine, respectively. These signals either directly or indirectly have effects on multiple transports that affect the secretory response as described in detail in the text. Adapted from Gorelick F, Pandol, SJ, Topazian M. *Pancreatic physiology, pathophysiology, acute and chronic pancreatitis.* Gastrointestinal Teaching Project, American Gastroenterologic Association. 2003.

lular negative electrical potential that drives negatively charged Cl^- and HCO_3^- secretion from the apical surface; the H^+-ATPase drives and Na^+/H^+ antiport facilitates formation of HCO_3^- from H_2O and CO_2 utilizing carbonic anhydrase; the Na^+/HCO_3^- cotransport provides additional intracellular HCO_3^- available for apical secretion. After transport of HCO_3^- into the ductal lumen, Na^+ and water are secreted into the ductal system to counter the electrical and osmotic forces resulting from the HCO_3^- secretion.

Of note, experimental data alone do not provide explanations for the ability of the pancreatic ductal system to secrete concentrations of $NaHCO_3$ as great as 140 mM. Mathematical modeling has been utilized in an attempt to show the relative roles of the known transporters to achieve such concentrations [4–6, 107]. One model [6] predicts that the only way to obtain such $NaHCO_3$ is to remove Cl^- from the system by preventing its entry through the basolateral membrane thus markedly decreasing its intracellular concentration. This model requires apical HCO_3^- secretion from the CFTR which it is capable of performing [105].

Although aspects of the pathways involved in $NaHCO_3$ and water are debated, the role of ion secretory pathways in maintaining normal exocrine pancreatic function is clear. Loss of function mutations in CFTR as occurs in cystic fibrosis results in severe exocrine pancreatic pathology with fibrosis of the gland associated with loss of exocrine pancreatic tissue. In fact, because patients with cystic fibrosis loose functional exocrine pancreatic tissue, they require lifelong treatment with oral preparations of commercially prepared digestive enzymes to digest meals and prevent malnutrition. These observations demonstrate the critical importance of the ion and water secretory pathways in maintenance of normal physiology.

In vitro experiments have demonstrated several agents that can inhibit ductal bicarbonate secretion [108]. These agents include methionine encephalin, insulin, somatostatin, peptide YY, substance P, basolaterally applied adenosine triphosphate, arginine vasopressin, 5-hydroxytryptamine and epidermal growth factor. The effects of substance P on inhibition of bicarbonate secretion are mediated by protein kinase C [109]. Although the physiologic role of these inhibitory agents is not known, some [108] speculate that the inhibition represents a protective mechanism stimulated by increased pressure in the pancreatic duct to attenuate the flow resulting in decreased pressure preventing potentially damaging effects of the increased pressure on the pancreas.

. . . .

Regulation of Whole-Organ Pancreatic Secretion

This section is devoted to describing the whole organ responses of the exocrine pancreas. Human exocrine pancreatic secretion occurs both during the fasting (interdigestive) state and after ingestion of a meal (digestive). The interdigestive pattern of secretion begins when the upper gastrointestinal tract is cleared of food. In an individual who eats three meals per day, the digestive pattern begins after breakfast and continues until late in the day, after the evening meal is cleared from the upper gastrointestinal tract.

INTERDIGESTIVE SECRETION

Interdigestive secretion is cyclic and follows the pattern of the migrating myoelectric complex (MMC) [110]. The patterns recur every 60 to 120 min, bursts of enzyme secretion being temporally associated with the periods of increased motor activity in the stomach and duodenum (i.e., phases II and III). In addition to pancreatic enzyme secretion, there is increased secretion of bicarbonate and bile (secondary to partial gallbladder contraction) into the duodenum during phases II and III of the MMC. The underlying mechanism involves the cholinergic nervous system [111]. The pancreatic secretion during the interdigestive phase is integral to the "housekeeping" function of the MMC to clear the small stomach and small intestine of debris including bacteria between meals [112].

DIGESTIVE SECRETION

The digestive secretion period is divided into three phases which are cephalic, gastric and intestinal. The reason for this division is that the network of regulatory systems responsible for effecting secretion shifts as a function of location of the meal and its effect on sensory inputs.

The *cephalic phase* of the meal represents the time before the swallowing of food and considers several stimuli that have inputs during this period. Such stimuli include emotional state, anticipation of the meal, auditory stimuli associated with the meal as well as the smell and taste of the meal and even chewing. The extent of cephalic stimulation of exocrine pancreatic secretion in humans has been evaluated through measurement of exocrine secretions stimulated by sham feeding (chewing and spitting out the food). The input from these sensory stimuli is integrated in the central nervous system nervous system at the dorsal vagal complex, and the output is transmitted to the exocrine pancreas via the vagus nerve.

Using sham feeding in humans, one study [113] demonstrated that sham feeding stimulated pancreatic enzyme secretion at up to 50% of the maximal secretory rate with no increase in bicarbonate secretion when gastric secretions were prevented from entering the duodenum. When gastric secretions were allowed entry into the duodenum, the rate of pancreatic enzyme secretion rose to about 90% of the maximal. With gastric secretions, entering bicarbonate was also secreted. These results suggest that cephalic stimulation specifically stimulates acinar secretion which has a low concentration of bicarbonate. When low pH gastric secretions are allowed to enter the duodenum, there was augmentation of both digestive enzyme and bicarbonate secretion from the pancreas. These results suggest that low pH in the duodenum from gastric secretions has effects on both acinar cell secretion (i.e., augmentation of digestive enzyme secretion) and ductal cell secretion (i.e., bicarbonate secretion). Of note, these effects of low pH in the duodenum are considered part of the gastric and intestinal phases of pancreatic secretion. Thus, the cephalic phase mediates secretion primarily from the acinar cell.

As indicated above, vagal efferents mediate the cephalic phase of pancreatic secretion. Because the acinar cell contains GPCRs for more than one neurotransmitter (i.e., acetylcholine, GRP, substance P, VIP), studies have been carried out to determine the relative roles of these neurotransmitters in mediating the secretory response of the acinar cell during the cephalic phase. Acetylcholine is certainly a major neurotransmitter involved because cholinergic antagonists greatly reduce and, in some cases, abolish sham feeding-stimulated pancreatic secretion in humans [114, 115]. Nerve endings containing the peptides VIP, GRP, CCK and enkephalins have been identified in the pancreas. Data supporting the role of these peptides in the cephalic phase of secretion are strongest for VIP and GRP [113, 116]. Both are released into the pancreatic venous effluent with vagal stimulation in animals. Furthermore, as discussed previously, acinar cells have GPCR receptors for GRP and VIP that mediate enzyme secretion.

The *gastric phase* of pancreatic secretion results from the effects of the meal in the stomach. The major stimulus of pancreatic secretion in the gastric phase is gastric distension [117], which causes predominantly secretion of digestive enzymes with little secretion of water and bicarbonate. That is, balloon distention of the stomach without nutrients present stimulates a low-volume, enzyme-rich secretion. The secretion is blocked by cholinergic inhibition, suggesting a gastropancreatic vagovagal reflex [117].

When gastric juice and contents of a meal enter the duodenum, a variety of intraluminal stimulants can act on the intestinal mucosa to stimulate pancreatic secretion through both neural and humoral mechanisms. Three gastric processes—secretion of acid, pepsin and lipase and emptying—are tightly coupled to the mechanisms of the intestinal phase of pancreatic secretion. Of note, salivary amylase also contributes to the digestion of starch and glycogen with the meal in the stomach. As indicated earlier, gastric acid entering the duodenum has an effect on both digestive enzyme secretion and bicarbonate secretion from the pancreas. Also, partial digestion of the protein, lipid and carbohydrate in the meal by pepsin, lipase and amylase, respectively, create nutrient stimulants that activate pancreatic secretion when delivered to the intestine. This discussion points out the interrelationship between the gastric phase and intestinal phase of the meal.

The *intestinal phase* of pancreatic secretion starts when chyme first enters the small intestine from the stomach and continues for the duration of the digestive period. It is mediated by both hormones and enteropancreatic vagovagal reflexes.

During the intestinal phase, the contribution of pancreatic ducts and their secretion of fluid with high concentrations of bicarbonate contribute significantly to the exocrine pancreatic output. The stimulant of this ductal secretion is hydrogen ion in the duodenum which causes the release of secretin from the secretin-containing S cell into the blood [118]. The secretin, in turn, interacts with its specific GPCRs on the pancreatic ductal cell to cause the fluid and bicarbonate secretion. Secretin is released from the basolateral surface of the S cell when the apical surface of the S cell which faces the lumen of the duodenum is exposed to gastric acid. The pH threshold for stimulation of secretin release into the blood is 4.5 [119–121]. The quantity of secretin released into the blood and the volume of pancreatic secretion are directly related to the load of titratable acid delivered to the duodenum. The role of secretin in meal-stimulated pancreatic fluid and bicarbonate secretion has been confirmed by showing that immune-neutralization of secretin with specific antisecretin antibody decreases these responses by as much as 80% [122, 123]. The antisecretin antibody also inhibits meal-stimulated enzyme secretion by as much as 50%, suggesting that secretin also has a role in enzyme secretion, possibly by potentiating the action of agonists, such as acetylcholine. These findings are consistent with those described earlier, showing that gastric acid stimulated during the cephalic phase that enters the duodenum increases fluid and bicarbonate secretion and augments pancreatic digestive enzyme secretion [113]. The results indicate that secretin plays key roles in regulating both ductal and acinar components of exocrine pancreatic secretion during a meal.

Of note, the bicarbonate response to secretin also depends on cholinergic input because atropine partially inhibits pancreatic bicarbonate secretion stimulated by intra-duodenal application of acid without an effect on the increase in blood concentration of secretin that occurs with the acid instillation [124, 125]. Furthermore, if exogenous secretin is infused to reproduce the plasma concentrations of secretin during a meal, the pancreatic bicarbonate output is less than the bicarbonate output observed with a meal. These results indicate that the bicarbonate and fluid response during a meal is mediated by a combination of cholinergic and hormonal secretin actions on the pancreatic ductal system.

Secretion of digestive enzymes during the intestinal phase is mediated by intraluminal fatty acids more than eight carbons in length, monoglycerides of these fatty acids, peptides, amino acids and, to a small extent, glucose [126–130]. The most potent amino acids for stimulating secretion in humans are phenylalanine, valine, methionine and tryptophan. The response to peptides and amino acids is related to the total load perfused into the intestine rather than the concentration. Importantly, digestion products of proteins, fats and carbohydrates are more effective stimulants of digestive enzyme secretion than the intact foodstuffs. These results indicate that secretion of digestive enzymes during the cephalic and gastric phases, as well as digestion occurring in the stomach, provides the stimuli for intestinal phase of pancreatic digestive enzyme secretion.

The pancreatic enzyme secretory response during the intestinal phase is mediated by both neural and hormonal pathways (Figure 15). Both removing the vagus nerve and administration of

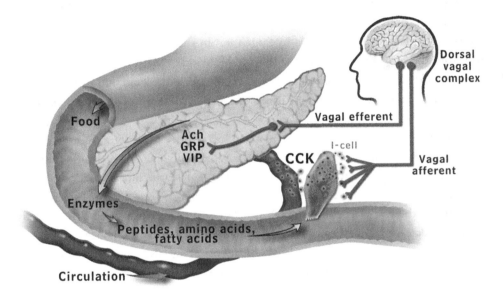

FIGURE 15: CCK stimulates pancreatic enzyme secretion by both neural and hormonal pathways. This cartoon shows the several pathways mediating meal-stimulated pancreatic secretion that involve CCK. First, meal nutrients, such as fatty acids, amino acids and peptides, delivered from the duodenum stimulate the release of CCK from the CCK-containing I cell to the area around the basolateral surface of the I cell. The CCK released can activate vagal afferent neurons that carry the signal to the dorsal vagal complex where the sensory information is integrated and vagal efferents are activated. Vagal efferents synapse with neurons in the pancreatic ganglia. In turn, via the neurotransmitters, acetylcholine (Ach), gastrin-releasing peptide (GRP) and vasoactive intestinal polypeptide (VIP) effector neurons in the pancreatic ganglia activate secretion by pancreatic acinar cells. In addition to activating the neural pathway, CCK released by the I cell enters the general circulation and may act as a hormone on the pancreatic acinar cells to cause secretion. Adapted from Gorelick F, Pandol, SJ, Topazian M. *Pancreatic physiology, pathophysiology, acute and chronic pancreatitis.* Gastrointestinal Teaching Project, American Gastroenterologic Association. 2003.

the cholinergic antagonist atropine markedly inhibit the digestive enzyme (and bicarbonate) responses to low intestinal loads of amino acids and fatty acids as well as infusion of physiologic concentrations of the hormone cholecystokinin (CCK) [131–134]. These results indicate a prominent role for the cholinergic nervous system utilizing vagovagal reflexes in the regulation of digestive enzyme secretion during the intestinal phase. Further, the results confirm a role for the cholinergic nervous system in bicarbonate secretion stimulated by secretin.

In addition to the role of neural pathways, the hormone CCK plays a major role in meal-stimulated digestive enzyme secretion during the intestinal phase. CCK concentrations in the blood increase during the intestinal phase of the meal with the main form being 58 amino acids in size (CCK-58) [127, 133, 135]. CCK is secreted from the basolateral surface of a specific endocrine cell in the mucosa of the upper small intestine called the I cell [136]. The apical surface of the I cell faces the lumen of the upper small intestine and releases CCK in response to digestion products of fat and protein and, to a lesser extent, by starch digestion products. Intravenous administration of CCK to provide blood concentrations achieved during a meal stimulates significant digestive enzyme secretion. In combination, these findings demonstrate that CCK is a key physiologic regulator of intestinal phase pancreatic digestive enzyme secretion.

The findings of key roles for both the cholinergic nervous system and CCK hormonal system in mediating digestive enzyme secretion have led to further investigations to determine potential interrelationships between the two systems. Resulting studies [133, 134] have demonstrated that CCK activates sensory afferent neurons in the duodenal mucosa. These afferent neurons activate a vagovagal reflex that causes pancreatic enzyme secretion (Figure 15). As indicated earlier, the pancreatic acinar cell has a functional CCK receptor that activates a digestive enzyme secretory response CCK [86]. Thus, the digestive enzyme secretory response to CCK can occur through direct hormonal activation of the acinar cell or indirectly through interacting with sensory neural afferents resulting in activation of a vagovagal reflex and direct cholinergic stimulation of the acinar cell.

INTESTINAL LUMINAL SENSORS INVOLVED IN PANCREATIC SECRETION

In the responses to the meal discussed above, little was mentioned about how the components of the meal are "sensed" resulting in activation of the regulatory pathways that mediate the pancreatic responses. The reason for describing the sensory machinery after the responses is that we know much less about the sensing mechanisms. The sensing that occurs during the cephalic phase of the meal involves olfactory and taste receptors. Although we know much less about sensing during the intestinal phase of the meal, research results are emerging indicating that the same taste receptors present on the tongue are represented throughout the intestine and that they are likely responsible for regulation of the neural and humoral pathways mediating pancreatic as well other gastrointestinal

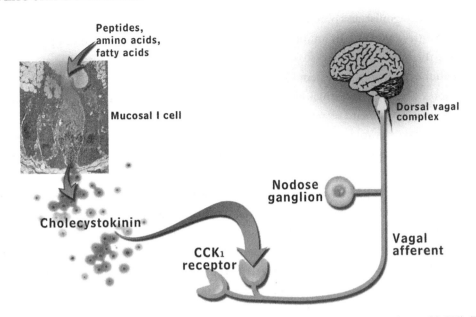

FIGURE 16: I cells "taste" intraluminal contents leading to release of cholecystokinin (CCK). The image is an electron photomicrograph of a CCK-secreting I cell. The I cell is one of the enterochromaffin cells. The apical surface of the I cell faces the lumen of the intestine where it "tastes" specific luminal nutrients (i.e., peptides, amino acids and fatty acids). As discussed in the text, the characterization of the sensors responding to intraluminal stimuli is under active investigation. When it senses the specific nutrients, the I cell is activated and releases CCK from its basal surface. CCK can either act as a hormone to circulate to the pancreas and stimulate a secretory response or interact with sensory afferents containing CCK A (also known as CCK_1) receptors. The image demonstrates the interaction of CCK with sensory receptors that are part of the enteric nervous system (ENS) of the gut. These neural receptors are located in proximity to the I cells. Vagal nerves to the CNS carry the afferent sensory signals. The afferent information going to the dorsal motor complex is processed and leads to stimulation of responses in the pancreas via vagal efferents. Adapted from Gorelick F, Pandol, SJ, Topazian M. *Pancreatic physiology, pathophysiology, acute and chronic pancreatitis.* Gastrointestinal Teaching Project, American Gastroenterologic Association. 2003.

responses [137–142]. Emerging information about taste receptors is more developed for humoral responses compared to neural responses.

The taste sensors are G-coupled protein receptors with a specific G coupling protein called Gαgustducin and respond to known tastant molecules [137, 139]. Several enteroendocrine cell types express TAS2R family bitter taste receptors and T1R2/3 sweet taste receptors [137, 139, 141–143].

As indicated earlier, the enteroendocrine cell I cell containing CCK and S cell containing secretin are present in the proximal intestine. These two cell types are representatives of many other enteroendocrine cells located throughout the gastrointestinal tract. Another prominent example includes the L cell in the more distal small intestine and proximal [144]. This cell contains glucagon-like peptide-1 (GLP-1) and peptide YY (PYY). The release of these hormones from each type of enteroendocrine cells is specific to the nutrient and/or environmental factors in the lumen of the gastrointestinal tract.

The electron micrograph in Figure 16 shows an I cell which is interspersed between non-endocrine intestinal epithelial cells. The I cells have microvilli facing the lumenal contents where they "taste" different nutrients in the lumenal stream. The basal portion of the I cell has vesicles containing CCK. When the I cell "tastes" specific nutrients like peptides, amino acids and/or fatty acids, the taste receptor activates an intracellular signaling system that activates calcium transients which, in turn, mediates the release of the CCK into the extracellular space at the base of the cell [145]. CCK can be taken up by the microvasculature and circulated to target tissues distant from the I cell. Also and importantly, CCK interacts with local sensory neurons containing specific receptors for CCK, as illustrated in Figure 15. Once activated, the neural pathways mediate many of the CCK functions. The afferent sensory pathways are carried by the vagus nerve, and the signals are received and integrated in the dorsal vagal complex (DVC) of the brain. Although not shown in the figure, efferent signals from the DVC then regulate pancreatic exocrine secretion as described earlier. Also, the efferent signals can regulate several other physiologic functions, including slowing gastric emptying of meal contents; contraction of the gallbladder; and relaxation of the sphincter that allows both gallbladder bile and pancreatic enzymes to enter into the lumen on the gut. These CCK-activated pathways also have a satiety effect resulting in decreased food intake.

FEEDBACK REGULATION OF PANCREATIC SECRETION

In both animals and humans, diversion of pancreatic secretions from the intestine results in augmented pancreatic secretion [146–149]. The mechanism of this effect of the pancreatic secretions has been of significant interest to physiologists and medical specialists in pancreatic diseases. The increase in digestive enzyme secretion with diversion is mediated by a rise in circulating CCK [148, 149]. Both the increase in circulating CCK and enzyme secretion occurring with diversion are prevented by intraluminal administration of trypsin and other protease digestive enzymes in humans [150]. These findings indicate that in addition to the mechanisms regulating pancreatic enzyme secretions described above during the cephalic, gastric and intestinal phases of the meal, there is feedback inhibitory regulation during the intestinal phase by the digestive enzymes themselves. Presumably, this inhibitory regulation modulates and fine tunes the amount of active digestive enzymes in the lumen of the intestine during the intestinal phase of the meal to ensure that there are sufficient amounts of digestive enzymes without excess provided for optimal rates of digestion. To accomplish this balance, it is hypothesized that during a meal, when trypsin (or other proteases) is occupied and is digesting meal proteins, pancreatic enzyme secretion is enhanced because trypsin is not available to interact with the surface of the intestine to cause the feedback inhibition. When there is excess digestive enzyme secretion and/or after digestion is complete, trypsin and other digestive proteases are free of the meal constituents and can interact directly with the intestinal luminal surface, resulting in inhibition of CCK release from the CCK-containing enteroendocrine I cell.

The mechanism of the digestive protease regulation of CCK release has been determined to involve intraluminal CCK-releasing factors. These releasing factors are hypothesized to play an intermediary role between the proteases and the I cell. Two proteins that can act as releasing factors have been described. One is called monitor peptide that is secreted by the pancreas into the lumen of the intestine [151]. The other is called luminal CCK-releasing factor (LCRF) that is present on the intestinal epithelium [152]. Both monitor peptide and LCRF cause CCK release from the I cell into the blood. These releasing factors are likely mediators of the physiologic feedback mechanism for enzyme secretion. It is believed that the effects of trypsin and other digestive enzymes are due to their ability to digest and inactivate monitor peptide and LCRF. Thus, in the presence of a meal when the digestive proteases are occupied, monitor peptide and LCRF interact with the I cell to promote CCK release and more digestive enzyme secretion. However, when there is an excess of digestive proteases in the intestinal lumen, both monitor peptide and LCRF are digested and inactivated so that their ability to augment CCK release and stimulate further pancreatic enzyme secretion ceases. In this way, the intraluminal processes that occur during the meal provide a fine-tuning mechanism to adjust the amount of digestive enzyme delivered to the meal for optimal rates of digestion.

Similar to the CCK-releasing factors, secretin-releasing factors have been described to regulate the release of secretin from the secretin-containing enteroendocrine S cell of the intestine [153, 154]. Phospholipase A_2 represents one secretin-releasing factor. Phospholipase A_2 is present in the mucosa of the upper small intestine and is released into the duodenum with intestinal acidification, and it causes secretin release into the circulation and stimulates a bicarbonate-rich pancreatic secretion with application to the upper small intestinal lumen. These results provide support for a secretin-releasing factor.

In addition to the proximal intestinal systems providing feedback regulation to the exocrine pancreas, there are also feedback regulatory systems in the distal small intestine. The most prominently studied one involves peptide YY (PYY) contained in endocrine cells of the distal small intestine [155–157]. PYY is released by administration of oleic acid into the lumen of the ilium. Circulating PYY inhibits CCK-stimulated pancreatic secretion through its effects on the area postrema of the brain leading the inhibitory regulation of vagal cholinergic mediation of pancreatic exocrine secretion.

·   ·   ·   ·

Measurement of Exocrine Pancreatic Secretion in Humans

Various measurement strategies have been developed to determine secretory function both for understanding normal physiology and determining the effects of disease states of the pancreas on secretory function [158–172]. These measurements of secretory function are divided into two groups: the direct measurements and the indirect measurements. Direct measurements of pancreatic secretory function involve collection of pancreatic secretions in the duodenum either without stimulation of the pancreas or after intravenous administration of a secretagogue or a combination of secretagogues combined with measurements of the ions and digestive enzymes in the secretions. Indirect measurements of pancreatic secretory function include the measurement of pancreatic enzymes in duodenal samples after nutrient ingestion, the measurement of products of digestive enzyme action on ingested substrates, and the measurement of pancreatic enzymes in the stool.

Which measurement to use depends on the physiologic or clinical question under consideration. A key point that has to be considered for any measurement strategy is that the exocrine pancreas has a large functional reserve. That is, the capacity for digestion is about 10 times of what is needed for complete digestion and absorption of a meal. Nutrient loss in the stool does not occur unless the functional capacity of the exocrine pancreas is less than 5% to 10% of normal as measured by CCK-stimulation of digestive enzyme secretion into the duodenum (a direct measurement technique) [126]. Thus, the indirect measurements that depend on the conversion of an ingested substrate to a measurable product will be insensitive to the changes in function that may occur in a disease state. Thus, the direct measurement of duodenal digestive enzymes, ions and water after the intravenous administration of pancreatic secretagogues provides the greatest sensitivity.

Direct measurements of pancreatic exocrine secretion are the most versatile for determining physiology during both interdigestive state and after administration of secretin, CCK or the two combined. The combination provides the complete information for both the acinar and ductular cell secretions. For this measurement, tubes are placed through the nose or mouth into both the stomach and duodenum for collection of secretions. The gastric tube is used to remove gastric secretions that would prevent the ability to measure water and bicarbonate secretion from the pancreas. The duodenal tube is used for collection of pancreatic secretions as well as delivering a nonabsorbable marker that can be used to determine the portion of the pancreatic secretions collected. For example, the use of a nonabsorbable marker, such as cobalamin or polyethylene glycol (PEG), allows the quantitation of secretions without the need for complete aspiration of secretions [161].

The direct measurements of pancreatic exocrine function are based on the principle that maximal water, bicarbonate and enzyme secretion are related to the functional mass of the pancreas [158, 159]. The intravenous administration of secretin, with volume and sodium bicarbonate measurement, provides information about the ductal function of the pancreas in normal states as well as various disease states. The intravenous administration of CCK and the measurement of digestive enzyme secretion have been used to successfully measure acinar cell function. Because the combination of secretin and CCK administration provides stimulation of both functional units of the exocrine pancreas, this combination is most commonly used [158, 159, 161–166]. CCK is best delivered by constant intravenous infusion. For measurements of maximal ductal secretion rates, synthetic secretin (SecroFlo, Repligen, Needham, MA) at a dose of 0.2 µg/kg injected over 1 minute is used. For maximal acinar secretion, synthetic CCK-octapeptide (carboxy-terminal octapeptide of CCK; Squibb, Princeton, NJ) at a dose of 40 ng/kg/h is used. Collections are made by aspiration of duodenal contents. Measurements, corrected for percentage recovery of the nonabsorbable marker, are made for fluid volume; bicarbonate and protein concentrations and the activity of various digestive enzymes (i.e., amylase, trypsin, chymotrypsin and lipase) [162].

More recently, a direct measurement method has been developed using endoscopy, and a short collection period has been described. An endoscopy which contains aspirating channels is passed into the duodenum [168–172]. Then, secretin, CCK or the combination of the two is administered intravenously, and pancreatic secretions are collected via the endoscope tip with its aspiration channel positioned in the duodenum.

The classic indirect measurement of pancreatic function with ingestion of a meal is the "Lundh Test Meal [160]." In the original description, the subject ingests a 300-mL liquid test meal composed of dried milk, vegetable oil and dextrose (6% fat, 5% protein and 15% carbohydrate). Samples are aspirated from the duodenum at intervals for measurement of digestive enzymes. The results of this type of measurement are dependent on the entire physiologic system, including the various sensory inputs during the different phases of the meal, the neurohumoral transmission systems and the pancreatic responses to the neurohumoral system. Thus, pancreatic enzyme secretory responses will be influenced by disorders of sensory organs, mucosal diseases of the upper intestine and alterations in the anatomy of the upper gastrointestinal tract. Comparisons of the results of the Lundh test meal (or variations of this meal) with those of direct measurement of pancreatic function can be used to show the influence of these factors on the pancreatic response [161].

There are several testing systems designed to measure of products of digestive enzyme action on ingested substrates. The most specific one is the measurement of stool triglyceride (also called stool fat or steatorrhea). Steatorrhea occurs when meal-stimulated pancreatic lipase output drops to less than 5% to 10% of normal [126]. For this measurement, the stools of the subject are collected for 72 h while he/she is ingesting a diet adequate in fat intake (70 to 100 g/day). Normally, 7% or less of ingested fat appears in the stool. A simple qualitative microscopic examination of a single stool for oil is almost as sensitive as quantitative measurements for fat [161]. Of note, this measurement is only useful in determining large losses of pancreatic function or significant alterations in anatomy or mucosal function because of the great amount of reserve of exocrine pancreatic function.

Several other indirect measurement systems have been designed that rely on digestive enzyme action on synthetic ingested substrates [161]. The substrates are acted upon by specific digestive enzymes, such as chymotrypsin and carboxylesterase, creating products that are measured in the urine, blood or breath. Again, because of the large functional reserve of the exocrine pancreas, these measurements are only able to determine large decreases in pancreatic secretory output. Finally, measurement of select pancreatic digestive enzymes, including chymotrypsin and elastase 1 in the stool, have been used to determine exocrine pancreatic insufficiency in patients with cystic fibrosis and chronic pancreatitis [173, 174].

. . . .

Clinical Application of Knowledge of Pancreatic Physiology

The understanding of the physiologic mechanisms involved in mediating pancreatic secretion during the intestinal phase of a meal can be utilized for clinical strategies. There are situations where it is necessary to provide nutrients to the intestinal tract of an individual without activating pancreatic secretions. One example occurs in patients with acute pancreatitis. This is a severe inflammatory disease of the exocrine pancreas that is made worse with stimulation of the exocrine pancreas [48]. This clinical need has led to investigations in humans to determine whether administration of alternative nutrients or delivery of nutrients to the jejunum rather than the duodenum may result in less activation of the pancreatic secretory response. Some examples are listed.

Studies in normal human volunteers compared the effect of equicaloric amounts of long fatty acid chain (long-chain) triglycerides and medium-chain triglycerides, infused into the jejunum, on plasma CCK levels and pancreatic secretion [175]. Long-chain triglycerides stimulated both an increase in CCK levels and pancreatic secretion while medium-chain triglycerides had no effect. Thus, with respect to jejunal administration, medium-chain triglycerides can be used to provide an energy source without significantly stimulating the pancreas.

Another study in healthy volunteers compared the effects of duodenal infusions of a complex liquid diet with those of an elemental (protein as amino acids) diet with low fat content [176]. Noteworthy was the finding of significantly less pancreatic secretion with the elemental diet than with the complex liquid diet. The combination of the findings in these two studies demonstrates that delivery of a diet with minimal need for digestion (i.e., elemental and medium-chain triglycerides) directly to the intestinal lumen bypassing the cephalic and gastric phases can provide nutrients with minimal stimulation of pancreatic secretions, an important strategy for providing nutrition to patients with acute pancreatitis.

Another clinical condition where application of knowledge of the mechanisms of pancreatic secretion has been used to develop treatments is chronic pancreatitis. Patients with this disorder have a chronic inflammatory and fibrosing process of the pancreas that is associated with constant and sometimes severe abdominal pain. Often, the pain is worsened with intake of a meal presumably due to stimulation of the pancreas. In some of these patients, oral administration of high doses of pancreatic enzymes alleviates the abdominal pain [177]. The mechanism of pain relief likely involves the feedback inhibition of pancreatic secretion discussed above.

·   ·   ·   ·

Summary

This chapter describes the multiple levels of regulation and coordination that are necessary for normal exocrine pancreatic function and digestion of a meal. For example, through independent and interacting neurohumoral pathways, a meal stimulates secretion of digestive enzymes from pancreatic acini and ions and water from the pancreatic duct cells into the duodenum. These secretory events require highly specialized cellular mechanisms that present unique opportunities for study of cellular physiology. This chapter also provides insights into the pathogenesis of pancreatic disorders as they relate to failure of cellular mechanisms responsible for key functions of the exocrine pancreas. Finally, and importantly, the chapter points out areas where information is lacking that is needed to both better understand the physiologic mechanisms and to provide potential opportunities for treatment of pancreatic diseases.

References

[1]   Bayliss, W.M., and Starling, E.H., The mechanism of pancreatic secretion. *J Physiol*, 1902. 28(5): pp. 325–53.

[2]   Palade, G., Intracellular aspects of the process of protein synthesis. *Science*, 1975. 189(4200): pp. 347–58.

[3]   Williams, J.A., Intracellular signaling mechanisms activated by cholecystokinin-regulating synthesis and secretion of digestive enzymes in pancreatic acinar cells. *Annu Rev Physiol*, 2001. 63: pp. 77–97.

[4]   Sohma, Y., et al., 150 mM HCO3(-)—how does the pancreas do it? Clues from computer modelling of the duct cell. *JOP*, 2001. 2(4 Suppl): pp. 198–202.

[5]   Steward, M.C., Ishiguro, H., and Case, R.M., Mechanisms of bicarbonate secretion in the pancreatic duct. *Annu Rev Physiol*, 2005. 67: pp. 377–409.

[6]   Whitcomb, D.C., and Ermentrout, G.B., A mathematical model of the pancreatic duct cell generating high bicarbonate concentrations in pancreatic juice. *Pancreas*, 2004. 29(2): pp. e30–40.

[7]   Ballian, N., and Brunicardi, F.C., Islet vasculature as a regulator of endocrine pancreas function. *World J Surg*, 2007. 31(4): pp. 705–14.

[8]   Korc, M., et al., Insulin action in pancreatic acini from streptozotocin-treated rats. I. Stimulation of protein synthesis. *Am J Physiol*, 1981. 240(1): pp. G56–62.

[9]   Korc, M., et al., Insulin receptors in isolated mouse pancreatic acini. *Biochem Biophys Res Commun*, 1978. 84(2): pp. 293–9.

[10]   Sankaran, H., et al., Insulin action in pancreatic acini from streptozotocin-treated rats. II. Binding of 125I-insulin to receptors. *Am J Physiol*, 1981. 240(1): pp. G63–8.

[11]   Muallem, S., et al., Actin filament disassembly is a sufficient final trigger for exocytosis in nonexcitable cells. *J Cell Biol*, 1995. 128(4): pp. 589–98.

[12]   O'Konski, M.S., and Pandol, S.J., Effects of caerulein on the apical cytoskeleton of the pancreatic acinar cell. *J Clin Invest*, 1990. 86(5): pp. 1649–57.

[13]   Fallon, M.B., et al., Effect of cerulein hyperstimulation on the paracellular barrier of rat exocrine pancreas. *Gastroenterology*, 1995. 108(6): pp. 1863–72.

[14] Stauffer, P.L., et al., Gap junction communication modulates [Ca2+]i oscillations and enzyme secretion in pancreatic acini. *J Biol Chem*, 1993. 268(26): pp. 19769–75.

[15] Yule, D.I., Stuenkel, E., and Williams, J.A. Intercellular calcium waves in rat pancreatic acini: mechanism of transmission. *Am J Physiol*, 1996. 271(4 Pt 1): pp. C1285–94.

[16] Omary, M.B., et al., The pancreatic stellate cell: a star on the rise in pancreatic diseases. *J Clin Invest*, 2007. 117(1): pp. 50–9.

[17] Pandol, S., et al., Desmoplasia of pancreatic ductal adenocarcinoma. *Clin Gastroenterol Hepatol*, 2009. 7(11 Suppl): pp. S44–7.

[18] Apte, M.V., Pirola, R.C., and Wilson, J.S., Battle-scarred pancreas: role of alcohol and pancreatic stellate cells in pancreatic fibrosis. *J Gastroenterol Hepatol*, 2006. 21(Suppl 3): pp. S97–101.

[19] Vonlaufen, A., et al., Pancreatic stellate cells and pancreatic cancer cells: an unholy alliance. *Cancer Res*, 2008. 68(19): pp. 7707–10.

[20] Bachem, M.G., et al., Pancreatic stellate cells—role in pancreas cancer. *Langenbecks Arch Surg*, 2008. 393(6): pp. 891–900.

[21] Bachem, M.G., et al., Role of stellate cells in pancreatic fibrogenesis associated with acute and chronic pancreatitis. *J Gastroenterol Hepatol*, 2006. 21(Suppl 3): pp. S92–6.

[22] Habener, J.F., Kemp, D.M., and, M.K. Thomas, Minireview: transcriptional regulation in pancreatic development. *Endocrinology*, 2005. 146(3): pp. 1025–34.

[23] Kim, S.K., and MacDonald, R.J., Signaling and transcriptional control of pancreatic organogenesis. *Curr Opin Genet Dev*, 2002. 12(5): pp. 540–7.

[24] Parkin, C.A., and Ingham, P.W., The adventures of Sonic Hedgehog in development and repair. I. Hedgehog signaling in gastrointestinal development and disease. *Am J Physiol Gastrointest Liver Physiol*, 2008. 294(2): p. G363–7.

[25] Kim, W., et al., Notch signaling in pancreatic endocrine cell and diabetes. *Biochem Biophys Res Commun*, 2010. 392(3): pp. 247–51.

[26] Case, R.M., Synthesis, intracellular transport and discharge of exportable proteins in the pancreatic acinar cell and other cells. *Biol Rev Camb Philos Soc*, 1978. 53(2): pp. 211–354.

[27] Petersen, O.H., and, A.V. Tepikin, Polarized calcium signaling in exocrine gland cells. *Annu Rev Physiol*, 2008. 70: pp. 273–99.

[28] Lingappa, V.R., and Blobel, G., Early events in the biosynthesis of secretory and membrane proteins: the signal hypothesis. *Recent Prog Horm Res*, 1980. 36: pp. 451–75.

[29] Simon, S.M., and Blobel, G., Mechanisms of translocation of proteins across membranes. *Subcell Biochem*, 1993. 21: pp. 1–15.

[30] Farquhar, M.G., and Palade, G.E., The Golgi apparatus: 100 years of progress and controversy. *Trends Cell Biol*, 1998. 8(1): pp. 2–10.

[31] Leitinger, B., Hille-Rehfeld, A., and Spiess, M., Biosynthetic transport of the asialoglyco-protein receptor H1 to the cell surface occurs via endosomes. *Proc Natl Acad Sci U S A*, 1995. 92(22): pp. 10109–13.

[32] Palade, G.E., Protein kinesis: the dynamics of protein trafficking and stability. Summary. *Cold Spring Harb Symp Quant Biol*, 1995. 60: pp. 821–31.

[33] Nemoto, T., et al., Stabilization of exocytosis by dynamic F-actin coating of zymogen granules in pancreatic acini. *J Biol Chem*, 2004. 279(36): pp. 37544–50.

[34] Poucell-Hatton, S., et al., Myosin I is associated with zymogen granule membranes in the rat pancreatic acinar cell. *Gastroenterology*, 1997. 113(2): pp. 649–58.

[35] Valentijn, J.A., et al., Actin coating of secretory granules during regulated exocytosis correlates with the release of rab3D. *Proc Natl Acad Sci U S A*, 2000. 97(3): pp. 1091–5.

[36] Hansen, N.J., Antonin, W., and Edwardson, J.M., Identification of SNAREs involved in regulated exocytosis in the pancreatic acinar cell. *J Biol Chem*, 1999. 274(32): pp. 22871–6.

[37] Ohnishi, H., et al., Involvement of Rab4 in regulated exocytosis of rat pancreatic acini. *Gastroenterology*, 1999. 116(4): pp. 943–52.

[38] Chen, X., et al., Rab27b localizes to zymogen granules and regulates pancreatic acinar exocytosis. *Biochem Biophys Res Commun*, 2004. 323(4): pp. 1157–62.

[39] Gaisano, H.Y., et al., Supramaximal cholecystokinin displaces Munc18c from the pancreatic acinar basal surface, redirecting apical exocytosis to the basal membrane. *J Clin Invest*, 2001. 108(11): pp. 1597–611.

[40] Cosen-Binker, L.I., et al., VAMP8 is the v-SNARE that mediates basolateral exocytosis in a mouse model of alcoholic pancreatitis. *J Clin Invest*, 2008. 118(7): pp. 2535–51.

[41] Ron, D., and Walter, P., Signal integration in the endoplasmic reticulum unfolded protein response. *Nat Rev Mol Cell Biol*, 2007. 8(7): pp. 519–29.

[42] Whitcomb, D.C., Genetic aspects of pancreatitis. *Annu Rev Med*, 2010. 61: pp. 413–24.

[43] Kereszturi, E., et al., Hereditary pancreatitis caused by mutation-induced misfolding of human cationic trypsinogen: a novel disease mechanism. *Hum Mutat*, 2009. 30(4): pp. 575–82.

[44] Lugea, A., et al., Adaptive unfolded protein response attenuates alcohol-induced pancreatic damage. *Gastroenterology*, 2010.

[45] Yadav, D., and Whitcomb, D.C., The role of alcohol and smoking in pancreatitis. *Nat Rev Gastroenterol Hepatol*, 2010. 7(3): pp. 131–45.

[46] Go, V.L., Gukovskaya, A., and S.J. Pandol, Alcohol and pancreatic cancer. *Alcohol*, 2005. 35(3): pp. 205–11.

[47] Maisonneuve, P., et al., Cigarette smoking accelerates progression of alcoholic chronic pancreatitis. *Gut*, 2005. 54(4): pp. 510–4.

[48]   Pandol, S.J., et al., Acute pancreatitis: bench to the bedside. *Gastroenterology*, 2007. 132(3): pp. 1127–51.

[49]   Rutkowski, D.T., and Kaufman, R.J., That which does not kill me makes me stronger: adapting to chronic ER stress. *Trends Biochem Sci*, 2007. 32(10): pp. 469–76.

[50]   Kim, I., Xu, W., and Reed, J.C., Cell death and endoplasmic reticulum stress: disease relevance and therapeutic opportunities. *Nat Rev Drug Discov*, 2008. 7(12): pp. 1013–30.

[51]   Marciniak, S.J., et al., Activation-dependent substrate recruitment by the eukaryotic translation initiation factor 2 kinase PERK. *J Cell Biol*, 2006. 172(2): pp. 201–9.

[52]   Kaser, A., et al., XBP1 links ER stress to intestinal inflammation and confers genetic risk for human inflammatory bowel disease. *Cell*, 2008. 134(5): pp. 743–56.

[53]   Yoshida, H., et al., XBP1 mRNA is induced by ATF6 and spliced by IRE1 in response to ER stress to produce a highly active transcription factor. *Cell*, 2001. 107(7): pp. 881–91.

[54]   Calfon, M., et al., IRE1 couples endoplasmic reticulum load to secretory capacity by processing the XBP-1 mRNA. *Nature*, 2002. 415(6867): pp. 92–6.

[55]   Lee, K., et al., IRE1-mediated unconventional mRNA splicing and S2P-mediated ATF6 cleavage merge to regulate XBP1 in signaling the unfolded protein response. *Genes Dev*, 2002. 16(4): pp. 452–66.

[56]   Yoshida, H., et al., A time-dependent phase shift in the mammalian unfolded protein response. *Dev Cell*, 2003. 4(2): pp. 265–71.

[57]   Shen, J., et al., ER stress regulation of ATF6 localization by dissociation of BiP/GRP78 binding and unmasking of Golgi localization signals. *Dev Cell*, 2002. 3(1): pp. 99–111.

[58]   Blais, J.D., et al., A small molecule inhibitor of endoplasmic reticulum oxidation 1 (ERO1) with selectively reversible thiol reactivity. *J Biol Chem*, 2010. 285(27): pp. 20993–1003.

[59]   Harding, H.P., et al., Regulated translation initiation controls stress-induced gene expression in mammalian cells. *Mol Cell*, 2000. 6(5): pp. 1099–108.

[60]   Scheuner, D., et al., Translational control is required for the unfolded protein response and in vivo glucose homeostasis. *Mol Cell*, 2001. 7(6): pp. 1165–76.

[61]   Harding, H.P., et al., An integrated stress response regulates amino acid metabolism and resistance to oxidative stress. *Mol Cell*, 2003. 11(3): pp. 619–33.

[62]   Oyadomari, S., and Mori, M., Roles of CHOP/GADD153 in endoplasmic reticulum stress. *Cell Death Differ*, 2004. 11(4): pp. 381–9.

[63]   Lowenfels, A.B., et al., Pancreatitis and the risk of pancreatic cancer. International Pancreatitis Study Group. *N Engl J Med*, 1993. 328(20): pp. 1433–7.

[64]   Scheele, G., Bartelt, D., and Bieger, W., Characterization of human exocrine pancreatic proteins by two-dimensional isoelectric focusing/sodium dodecyl sulfate gel electrophoresis. *Gastroenterology*, 1981. 80(3): pp. 461–73.

[65]   Beck, I.T., The role of pancreatic enzymes in digestion. *Am J Clin Nutr*, 1973. 26(3): pp. 311–25.

[66]   Whitcomb, D.C., and Lowe, M.E., Human pancreatic digestive enzymes. *Dig Dis Sci*, 2007. 52(1): pp. 1–17.

[67]   Rinderknecht, H., Activation of pancreatic zymogens. Normal activation, premature intra-pancreatic activation, protective mechanisms against inappropriate activation. *Dig Dis Sci*, 1986. 31(3): pp. 314–21.

[68]   Pubols, M.H., Bartelt, D.C., and Greene, L.J., Trypsin inhibitor from human pancreas and pancreatic juice. *J Biol Chem*, 1974. 249(7): pp. 2235–42.

[69]   Gorry, M.C., et al., Mutations in the cationic trypsinogen gene are associated with recurrent acute and chronic pancreatitis. *Gastroenterology*, 1997. 113(4): pp. 1063–8.

[70]   Whitcomb, D.C., et al., Hereditary pancreatitis is caused by a mutation in the cationic trypsinogen gene. *Nat Genet*, 1996. 14(2): pp. 141–5.

[71]   Meites, S., and Rogols, S., Amylase isoenzymes. *CRC Crit Rev Clin Lab Sci*, 1971. 2(1): pp. 103–38.

[72]   Kimmich, G.A., Membrane potentials and the mechanism of intestinal Na(+)-dependent sugar transport. *J Membr Biol*, 1990. 114(1): pp. 1–27.

[73]   Wright, E.M., Martin, M.G., and Turk, E., Intestinal absorption in health and disease—sugars. *Best Pract Res Clin Gastroenterol*, 2003. 17(6): pp. 943–56.

[74]   Hofmann, A.F., and Borgstrom, B., Hydrolysis of long-chain monoglycerides in micellar solution by pancreatic lipase. *Biochim Biophys Acta*, 1963. 70: p. 317–31.

[75]   Kilberg, M.S., Stevens, B.R., and Novak, D.A., Recent advances in mammalian amino acid transport. *Annu Rev Nutr*, 1993. 13: pp. 137–65.

[76]   Boulet, A.M., Erwin, C.R., and Rutter, W.J., Cell-specific enhancers in the rat exocrine pancreas. *Proc Natl Acad Sci U S A*, 1986. 83(11): pp. 3599–603.

[77]   Cockell, M., et al., Identification of a cell-specific DNA-binding activity that interacts with a transcriptional activator of genes expressed in the acinar pancreas. *Mol Cell Biol*, 1989. 9(6): pp. 2464–76.

[78]   Stevenson, B.J., Hagenbuchle, O., and Wellauer, P.K., Sequence organisation and transcriptional regulation of the mouse elastase II and trypsin genes. *Nucleic Acids Res*, 1986. 14(21): pp. 8307–30.

[79]   Howard, G., et al., Binding of a pancreatic nuclear protein is correlated with amylase enhancer activity. *Nucleic Acids Res*, 1989. 17(20): pp. 8185–95.

[80]   Keller, S.A., et al., Regulation of amylase gene expression in diabetic mice is mediated by a cis-acting upstream element close to the pancreas-specific enhancer. *Genes Dev*, 1990. 4(8): pp. 1316–21.

[81]   Kruse, F., et al., Cooperation between elements of an organ-specific transcriptional en-
       hancer in animals. *Mol Cell Biol*, 1995. 15(8): pp. 4385–94.

[82]   Rose, S.D., et al., A single element of the elastase I enhancer is sufficient to direct transcrip-
       tion selectively to the pancreas and gut. *Mol Cell Biol*, 1994. 14(3): pp. 2048–57.

[83]   Brannon, P.M., Adaptation of the exocrine pancreas to diet. *Annu Rev Nutr*, 1990. 10:
       pp. 85–105.

[84]   Birk, R.Z., et al., Pancreatic lipase and its related protein 2 are regulated by dietary
       polyunsaturated fat during the postnatal development of rats. *Pediatr Res*, 2004. 56(2):
       pp. 256–62.

[85]   Perkins, P.S., Rutherford, R.E., and Pandol, S.J., Effect of chronic ethanol feeding on diges-
       tive enzyme synthesis and mRNA content in rat pancreas. *Pancreas*, 1995. 10(1): pp. 14–21.

[86]   Murphy, J.A., et al., Direct activation of cytosolic Ca2+ signaling and enzyme secretion by
       cholecystokinin in human pancreatic acinar cells. *Gastroenterology*, 2008. 135(2): pp. 632–41.

[87]   Williams, J.A., Regulation of acinar cell function in the pancreas. *Curr Opin Gastroenterol*,
       2010. 26(5): pp. 478–83.

[88]   Wank, S.A., G protein-coupled receptors in gastrointestinal physiology. I. CCK receptors:
       an exemplary family. *Am J Physiol*, 1998. 274(4 Pt 1): pp. G607–13.

[89]   Williams, J.A., Regulation of pancreatic acinar cell function. *Curr Opin Gastroenterol*, 2006.
       22(5): pp. 498–504.

[90]   Petersen, O.H., Petersen, C.C., and Kasai, H., Calcium and hormone action. *Annu Rev
       Physiol*, 1994. 56: p. 297–319.

[91]   Kasai, H., and Petersen, O.H., Spatial dynamics of second messengers: IP3 and cAMP as
       long-range and associative messengers. *Trends Neurosci*, 1994. 17(3): pp. 95–101.

[92]   Kasai, H., Li, Y.X., and Miyashita, Y., Subcellular distribution of Ca2+ release channels un-
       derlying Ca2+ waves and oscillations in exocrine pancreas. *Cell*, 1993. 74(4): pp. 669–77.

[93]   Maruyama, Y., et al., Agonist-induced localized Ca2+ spikes directly triggering exocytotic
       secretion in exocrine pancreas. *EMBO J*, 1993. 12(8): pp. 3017–22.

[94]   Fitzsimmons, T.J., et al., Acyl-coenzyme A causes Ca2+ release in pancreatic acinar cells.
       J Biol Chem, 1997. 272(50): pp. 31435–40.

[95]   Pandol, S.J., et al., Role of free cytosolic calcium in secretagogue-stimulated amylase release
       from dispersed acini from guinea pig pancreas. *J Biol Chem*, 1985. 260(18): pp. 10081–6.

[96]   Bahnson, T.D., Pandol, S.J., and Dionne, V.E., Cyclic GMP modulates depletion-activated
       Ca2+ entry in pancreatic acinar cells. *J Biol Chem*, 1993. 268(15): pp. 10808–12.

[97]   Lee, K.P., et al., An endoplasmic reticulum/plasma membrane junction: STIM1/Orai1/
       TRPCs. [*FEBS Lett*, 2010. 584(10): pp. 2022–7.

[98]   Parekh, A.B., Store-operated CRAC channels: function in health and disease. *Nat Rev Drug Discov*, 2010. 9(5): pp. 399–410.

[99]   Sutton, R., Petersen, O.H., and Pandol, S.J., Pancreatitis and calcium signalling: report of an international workshop. *Pancreas*, 2008. 36(4): pp. e1–14.

[100] Pandol, S.J., et al., Dual pathways for agonist-stimulated arachidonic acid release in pancreatic acini: roles in secretion. *Am J Physiol*, 1991. 260(3 Pt 1): pp. G423–33.

[101] Pandol, S.J., and Schoeffield, M.S., 1,2-Diacylglycerol, protein kinase C, and pancreatic enzyme secretion. *J Biol Chem*, 1986. 261(10): pp. 4438–44.

[102] Nishimori, I., and Onishi, S., Carbonic anhydrase isozymes in the human pancreas. *Dig Liver Dis*, 2001. 33(1): pp. 68–74.

[103] Nishimori, I., et al., Carbonic anhydrase in human pancreas: hypotheses for the pathophysiological roles of CA isozymes. *Ann N Y Acad Sci*, 1999. 880: pp. 5–16.

[104] Marino, C.R., et al., Localization of the cystic fibrosis transmembrane conductance regulator in pancreas. *J Clin Invest*, 1991. 88(2): pp. 712–6.

[105] Ishiguro, H., et al., CFTR functions as a bicarbonate channel in pancreatic duct cells. *J Gen Physiol*, 2009. 133(3): pp. 315–26.

[106] Stuenkel, E.L., Machen, T.E., and Williams, J.A., pH regulatory mechanisms in rat pancreatic ductal cells. *Am J Physiol*, 1988. 254(6 Pt 1): pp. G925–30.

[107] Sohma, Y., et al., HCO_3—transport in a mathematical model of the pancreatic ductal epithelium. *J Membr Biol*, 2000. 176(1): pp. 77–100.

[108] Hegyi, P., and Rakonczay, Z. Jr., The inhibitory pathways of pancreatic ductal bicarbonate secretion. *Int J Biochem Cell Biol*, 2007. 39(1): pp. 25–30.

[109] Hegyi, P., et al., Protein kinase C mediates the inhibitory effect of substance P on HCO3- secretion from guinea pig pancreatic ducts. *Am J Physiol Cell Physiol*, 2005. 288(5): pp. C1030–41.

[110] DiMagno, E.P., et al., Relationships among canine fasting pancreatic and biliary secretions, pancreatic duct pressure, and duodenal phase III motor activity—Boldyreff revisited. *Dig Dis Sci*, 1979. 24(9): pp. 689–93.

[111] Zimmerman, D.W., et al., Cyclic interdigestive pancreatic exocrine secretion: is it mediated by neural or hormonal mechanisms? *Gastroenterology*, 1992. 102(4 Pt 1): pp. 1378–84.

[112] Otterson, M.F., and Sarr, M.G., Normal physiology of small intestinal motility. *Surg Clin North Am*, 1993. 73(6): pp. 1173–92.

[113] Anagnostides, A., et al., Sham feeding and pancreatic secretion. Evidence for direct vagal stimulation of enzyme output. *Gastroenterology*, 1984. 87(1): pp. 109–14.

[114] Katschinski, M., et al., Cephalic stimulation of gastrointestinal secretory and motor responses in humans. *Gastroenterology*, 1992. 103(2): pp. 383–91.

[115] Katschinski, M., et al., Gastrointestinal motor and secretory responses to cholinergic stimulation in humans. Differential modulation by muscarinic and cholecystokinin receptor blockade. *Eur J Clin Invest*, 1995. 25(2): pp. 113–22.

[116] Holst, J.J., et al., Interrelation of nerves and hormones in stomach and pancreas. *Scand J Gastroenterol Suppl*, 1983. 82: pp. 85–99.

[117] Kreiss, C., et al., Role of antrum in regulation of pancreaticobiliary secretion in humans. *Am J Physiol*, 1996. 270(5 Pt 1): pp. G844–51.

[118] Konturek, S.J., Dubiel, J., and Gabrys, B., Effect of acid infusion into various levels of the intestine on gastric and pancreatic secretion in the cat. *Gut*, 1969. 10(9): pp. 749–53.

[119] Chey, W.Y., and Konturek, S.J., Plasma secretion and pancreatic secretion in response to liver extract meal with varied pH and exogenous secretin in the dog. *J Physiol*, 1982. 324: pp. 263–72.

[120] Meyer, J.H., Way, L.W., and Grossman, M.I., Pancreatic bicarbonate response to various acids in duodenum of the dog. *Am J Physiol*, 1970. 219(4): pp. 964–70.

[121] Meyer, J.H., Way, L.W., and Grossman, M.I., Pancreatic response to acidification of various lengths of proximal intestine in the dog. *Am J Physiol*, 1970. 219(4): pp. 971–7.

[122] Chey, W.Y., et al., Effect of rabbit antisecretin serum on postprandial pancreatic secretion in dogs. *Gastroenterology*, 1979. 77(6): pp. 1268–75.

[123] Song, Y., et al., Canine pancreatic juice stimulates the release of secretin and pancreatic secretion in the dog. *Am J Physiol*, 1999. 277(3 Pt 1): pp. G731–5.

[124] You, C.H., Rominger, J.M., and Chey, W.Y., Effects of atropine on the action and release of secretin in humans. *Am J Physiol*, 1982. 242(6): pp. G608–11.

[125] Singer, M.V., et al., Effect of atropine on pancreatic response to HCl and secretin. *Am J Physiol*, 1981. 240(5): pp. G376–80.

[126] Go, V.L., Hofmann, A.F., and Summerskill, W.H., Pancreozymin bioassay in man based on pancreatic enzyme secretion: potency of specific amino acids and other digestive products. *J Clin Invest*, 1970. 49(8): pp. 1558–64.

[127] Liddle, R.A., et al., Cholecystokinin bioactivity in human plasma. Molecular forms, responses to feeding, and relationship to gallbladder contraction. *J Clin Invest*, 1985. 75(4): pp. 1144–52.

[128] Meyer, J.H., and Kelly, G.A., Canine pancreatic responses to intestinally perfused proteins and protein digests. *Am J Physiol*, 1976. 231(3): pp. 682–91.

[129] Meyer, J.H., et al., Canine gut receptors mediating pancreatic responses to luminal L-amino acids. *Am J Physiol*, 1976. 231(3): pp. 669–77.

[130] Meyer, J.H., Kelly, G.A., and Jones, R.S., Canine pancreatic response to intestinally perfused oligopeptides. *Am J Physiol*, 1976. 231(3): pp. 678–81.

[131] Singer, M.V., Solomon, T.E., and Grossman, M.I., Effect of atropine on secretion from intact and transplanted pancreas in dog. *Am J Physiol*, 1980. 238(1): pp. G18–22.

[132] Singer, M.V., et al., Pancreatic secretory response to intravenous caerulein and intraduodenal tryptophan studies: before and after stepwise removal of the extrinsic nerves of the pancreas in dogs. *Gastroenterology*, 1989. 96(3): pp. 925–34.

[133] Owyang, C., Physiological mechanisms of cholecystokinin action on pancreatic secretion. *Am J Physiol*, 1996. 271(1 Pt 1): pp. G1–7.

[134] Li, Y., Hao, Y, and Owyang, C., High-affinity CCK-A receptors on the vagus nerve mediate CCK-stimulated pancreatic secretion in rats. *Am J Physiol*, 1997. 273(3 Pt 1): pp. G679–85.

[135] Reeve, J.R., Jr., et al., CCK-58 is the only detectable endocrine form of cholecystokinin in rat. *Am J Physiol Gastrointest Liver Physiol*, 2003. 285(2): pp. G255–65.

[136] Liddle, R.A., Cholecystokinin cells. *Annu Rev Physiol*, 1997. 59: pp. 221–42.

[137] Rozengurt, E., Taste receptors in the gastrointestinal tract. I. Bitter taste receptors and alpha-gustducin in the mammalian gut. *Am J Physiol Gastrointest Liver Physiol*, 2006. 291(2): pp. G171–7.

[138] Rozengurt, E., and Sternini, C., Taste receptor signaling in the mammalian gut. *Curr Opin Pharmacol*, 2007. 7(6): pp. 557–62.

[139] Sternini, C., Anselmi, L., and Rozengurt, E. Enteroendocrine cells: a site of 'taste' in gastrointestinal chemosensing. *Curr Opin Endocrinol Diabetes Obes*, 2008. 15(1): pp. 73–8.

[140] Dyer, J., et al., Intestinal glucose sensing and regulation of intestinal glucose absorption. *Biochem Soc Trans*, 2007. 35(Pt 5): pp. 1191–4.

[141] Dyer, J., et al., Expression of sweet taste receptors of the T1R family in the intestinal tract and enteroendocrine cells. *Biochem Soc Trans*, 2005. 33(Pt 1): pp. 302–5.

[142] Margolskee, R.F., et al., T1R3 and gustducin in gut sense sugars to regulate expression of Na+-glucose cotransporter 1. *Proc Natl Acad Sci U S A*, 2007. 104(38): pp. 15075–80.

[143] Wu, S.V., et al., Expression of bitter taste receptors of the T2R family in the gastrointestinal tract and enteroendocrine STC-1 cells. *Proc Natl Acad Sci U S A*, 2002. 99(4): pp. 2392–7.

[144] Rozengurt, N., et al., Colocalization of the alpha-subunit of gustducin with PYY and GLP-1 in L cells of human colon. *Am J Physiol Gastrointest Liver Physiol*, 2006. 291(5): pp. G792–802.

[145] Chen, M.C., et al., Bitter stimuli induce Ca2+ signaling and CCK release in enteroendocrine STC-1 cells: role of L-type voltage-sensitive Ca2+ channels. *Am J Physiol Cell Physiol*, 2006. 291(4): pp. C726–39.

[146] Green, G.M., and, Lyman, R.L. Chymotrypsin inhibitor stimulation of pancreatic enzyme secretion in the rat. *Proc Soc Exp Biol Med*, 1971. 136(2): pp. 649–54.

[147] Green, G.M., and Lyman, R.L. Feedback regulation of pancreatic enzyme secretion as a

mechanism for trypsin inhibitor-induced hypersecretion in rats. *Proc Soc Exp Biol Med*, 1972. 140(1): pp. 6–12.

[148] Louie, D.S., et al., Cholecystokinin mediates feedback regulation of pancreatic enzyme secretion in rats. *Am J Physiol*, 1986. 250(2 Pt 1): pp. G252–9.

[149] Owyang, C., Louie, D.S., and Tatum, D. Feedback regulation of pancreatic enzyme secretion. Suppression of cholecystokinin release by trypsin. *J Clin Invest*, 1986. 77(6): pp. 2042–7.

[150] Walkowiak, J., et al., Inhibition of endogenous pancreatic enzyme secretion by oral pancreatic enzyme treatment. *Eur J Clin Invest*, 2003. 33(1): pp. 65–9.

[151] Liddle, R.A., Regulation of cholecystokinin secretion by intraluminal releasing factors. *Am J Physiol*, 1995. 269(3 Pt 1): pp. G319–27.

[152] Spannagel, A.W., et al., Purification and characterization of a luminal cholecystokinin-releasing factor from rat intestinal secretion. *Proc Natl Acad Sci U S A*, 1996. 93(9): pp. 4415–20.

[153] Li, J.P., et al., Pancreatic phospholipase A2 from the small intestine is a secretin-releasing factor in rats. *Am J Physiol Gastrointest Liver Physiol*, 2001. 281(2): pp. G526–32.

[154] Chang, T.M., et al., Purification of two secretin-releasing peptides structurally related to phospholipase A2 from canine pancreatic juice. *Pancreas*, 1999. 19(4): pp. 401–5.

[155] Naruse, S., et al., Feedback regulation of pancreatic secretion by peptide YY. *Peptides*, 2002. 23(2): pp. 359–65.

[156] Teyssen, S., et al., Inhibition of canine exocrine pancreatic secretion by peptide YY is mediated by PYY-preferring Y2 receptors. *Pancreas*, 1996. 13(1): pp. 80–8.

[157] Deng, X., et al., PYY inhibits CCK-stimulated pancreatic secretion through the area postrema in unanesthetized rats. *Am J Physiol Regul Integr Comp Physiol*, 2001. 281(2): pp. R645–53.

[158] Hansky, J., et al., Relationship between maximal secretory output and weight of the pancreas in the dog. *Proc Soc Exp Biol Med*, 1963. 114: pp. 654–6.

[159] Hansky, J., et al., Maximal secretory capacity of the canine pancreas in response to pancreozymin and secretin. *Am J Physiol*, 1964. 206: pp. 351–6.

[160] Lundh, G., Pancreatic exocrine function in neoplastic and inflammatory disease; a simple and reliable new test. *Gastroenterology*, 1962. 42: pp. 275–80.

[161] Niederau, C., and Grendell, J.H., Diagnosis of chronic pancreatitis. *Gastroenterology*, 1985. 88(6): pp. 1973–95.

[162] Boyd, E.J., Rinderknecht, H., and Wormsley, K.G., Laboratory tests in the diagnosis of the chronic pancreatic diseases. Part 4. Tests involving the measurement of pancreatic enzymes in body fluid. *Int J Pancreatol*, 1988. 3(1): pp. 1–16.

[163] Boyd, E.J., Rinderknecht, H., and Wormsley, K.G., Laboratory tests in the diagnosis of

the chronic pancreatic diseases. Part 6. Differentiation between chronic pancreatitis and pancreatic cancer. *Int J Pancreatol*, 1988. 3(4): pp. 229–40.

[164] Boyd, E.J., and Wormsley, K.G., Laboratory tests in the diagnosis of the chronic pancreatic diseases. Part 1. Secretagogues used in tests of pancreatic secretion. *Int J Pancreatol*, 1987. 2(3): pp. 137–48.

[165] Boyd, E.J., and Wormsley, K.G., Laboratory tests in the diagnosis of the chronic pancreatic diseases. Part 2. Tests of pancreatic secretion. *Int J Pancreatol*, 1987. 2(4): pp. 211–21.

[166] Boyd, E.J., and Wormsley, K.G., Laboratory tests in the diagnosis of the chronic pancreatic diseases. Part 5. Stool enzyme measurements. *Int J Pancreatol*, 1988. 3(2–3): pp. 101–3.

[167] Rinderknecht, H., Boyd, E.J., and Wormsley, K.G., Laboratory tests in the diagnosis of the chronic pancreatic diseases. Part 3. Tests on pure pancreatic juice. *Int J Pancreatol*, 1987. 2(5–6): pp. 291–304.

[168] Conwell, D.L., et al., Analysis of duodenal drainage fluid after cholecystokinin (CCK) stimulation in healthy volunteers. *Pancreas*, 2002. 25(4): pp. 350–4.

[169] Conwell, D.L., et al., An endoscopic pancreatic function test with cholecystokinin-octapeptide for the diagnosis of chronic pancreatitis. *Clin Gastroenterol Hepatol*, 2003. 1(3): pp. 189–94.

[170] Stevens, T., et al., Electrolyte composition of endoscopically collected duodenal drainage fluid after synthetic porcine secretin stimulation in healthy subjects. *Gastrointest Endosc*, 2004. 60(3): pp. 351–5.

[171] Wu, B., and Conwell, D.L., The endoscopic pancreatic function test. *Am J Gastroenterol*, 2009. 104(10): pp. 2381–3.

[172] Raimondo, M., Imoto, M., and DiMagno, E.P., Rapid endoscopic secretin stimulation test and discrimination of chronic pancreatitis and pancreatic cancer from disease controls. *Clin Gastroenterol Hepatol*, 2003. 1(5): pp. 397–403.

[173] Borowitz, D., Update on the evaluation of pancreatic exocrine status in cystic fibrosis. *Curr Opin Pulm Med*, 2005. 11(6): pp. 524–7.

[174] Daftary, A., et al., Fecal elastase-1: utility in pancreatic function in cystic fibrosis. *J Cyst Fibros*, 2006. 5(2): pp. 71–6.

[175] Symersky, T., et al., The effect of equicaloric medium-chain and long-chain triglycerides on pancreas enzyme secretion. *Clin Physiol Funct Imaging*, 2002. 22(5): pp. 307–11.

[176] O'Keefe, S.J., et al., Physiological effects of enteral and parenteral feeding on pancreaticobiliary secretion in humans. *Am J Physiol Gastrointest Liver Physiol*, 2003. 284(1): pp. G27–36.

[177] Gupta, V., and Toskes, P.P., Diagnosis and management of chronic pancreatitis. *Postgrad Med J*, 2005. 81(958): pp. 491–7.